Praise for *Love Your Bones*

'One of the most shocking photog my mother's spine. It was almos watched her stooped shoulders and bent position from which she could never rise. Nor If, as Max Tuck says, "this is a whole body we live in" it is no good fixing a puncture if the steering is broken as well.

'There may be many books written on the subject of osteoporosis, but this one is different. Refreshingly so.'

Virginia McKenna OBE
Actress, author and wildlife campaigner

'Max has a gift to create real clarity around the subject of nutrition and her passion shines through with this book. For any of you that really care about your health, and want to take control of your body's strength for the future, then this is the book for you. With her unbelievable knowledge about nutrition and health, this book gives you the most up-to-date and correct information, which would take most people years to research. It is clear that Max wants to share this knowledge to give everyone a chance to change, improve and gain understanding to create the best, most vibrant life possible. It is brilliantly written and explained, and I certainly will be recommending it to all my clients. Knowledge is power!'

Denise Kelly
Naturopathic Nutritional Therapist; Director, Denise Kelly Nutrition

'Max Tuck is one of the UK's leading experts on health and nutrition, and a shining example of what she teaches. If you want to protect your bones while also enhancing every aspect of your health and wellbeing (and to do all of that the raw vegan way) get your copy of this gem of a book, and follow her recommendations.'

Sarah Best
Nutritionist, author and health coach

'It is always an absolute pleasure to host Max on *Food for Thought* and *Natural Health Radio*. She's considered one of our expert speakers on nutrition, who is a firm favourite with the listeners. Why? Because she knows her subject inside out, gets straight to the point, is absolutely no-nonsense, as well as being very well-researched with the latest findings. She's a woman who shows her passion about health, and understands how nature balances and heals the body.

'The message about bone health in the mainstream media is mostly aimed at women, yet men also have to deal with this increasing health problem, caused largely by diet and lifestyle issues. Max absolutely comprehends this and her knowledge helps you to future-proof yourself with diet and lifestyle changes.'

Deborah Walker
Naturopathic Nutritionist and Founder of Natural Health Radio

'Max is the busiest person I know, combining her high-pressure work in a large veterinary practice with an ever-expanding nutritional consultancy; teaching courses, running retreats, giving lectures, writing articles and newsletters, keeping her website up to date, writing books and maintaining her fantastic state of health and fitness with an incredible exercise regime and the perfect plant-based diet. She absolutely leads by example.

'With a wealth of information at her fingertips, Max explains with extraordinary clarity and great humour the well-researched, scientifically proven facts concerning bone health, nutrition and fitness. She is a mine of knowledge and practical advice.

'Follow Max's advice and her shining example and you cannot help but enjoy abundant health, energy and vitality.'

Susanna McIntyre BVSc, MRCVS, PDNN
Founding President, BVDA

'Max Tuck is one of the most informative and knowledgeable speakers that I have met. She takes her passion for health and nutrition and funnels it through the pages of this book. Recommended!'

Philip McCluskey
Author and motivational speaker, life coach

'Although this book is called 'Love Your Bones', don't be fooled! Max has synthesized the most cutting-edge principles, strategies and wisdom to set you free and allow you to experience phenomenal health. Max walks her talk more than anyone I know, you'll love her story and personal journey, and to top it all off she has proved the principles work. Also, having known Max for many years, I know her standards are as high as they come, her integrity is second to none, and with that you'd be crazy not to read and master this phenomenal book.'

Mike Nash
Director, Raw Perfection Ltd; Author, Aggressive Health

LOVE YOUR BONES

The essential guide to ending osteoporosis and building a healthy skeleton

This book is dedicated to Jean Tuck, my mother and fellow Capricorn, whose diagnosis of osteoporosis led me to start researching this epidemic that is sweeping through the Western world.

LOVE YOUR BONES

The essential guide to ending osteoporosis and building a healthy skeleton

Max Tuck
aka The Raw Food Scientist

with a Foreword by
Brian R. Clement
Director, Hippocrates Health Institute, Florida, USA

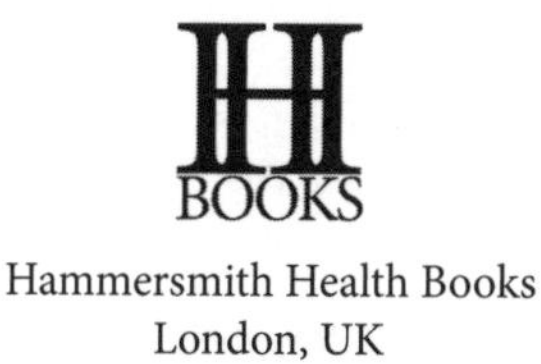

Hammersmith Health Books
London, UK

First published in 2015 by Hammersmith Health Books – an imprint of Hammersmith Books Limited
14 Greville Street, London EC1N 8SB, UK
www.hammersmithbooks.co.uk

Disclaimer: The information contained in this book is for educational purposes only. It is the result of the study and the experience of the author. Whilst the information and advice offered are believed to be true and accurate at the time of going to press, neither the author nor the publisher can accept any legal responsibility or liability for any errors or omissions that may have been made or for any adverse effects which may occur as a result of following the recommendations given herein. Always consult a qualified medical practitioner if you have any concerns regarding your health.

British Library Cataloguing in Publication Data: A CIP record of this book is available from the British Library.

Print ISBN 978-1-78161-071-8
Ebook ISBN 978-1-78161-072-5

Commissioning editor: Georgina Bentliff
Designed and typeset by: Julie Bennett, Bespoke Publishing Ltd
Cover design by: Julie Bennett
Index: Dr Laurence Errington
Production: Helen Whitehorn, Path Projects Ltd
Printed and bound by: TJ International Ltd, Cornwall, UK

Contents

Foreword

Dr Max Tuck possesses the experience, intuition and common sense to present this brilliant publication. Over the years, I have observed her enthusiastically reaching for new and cutting-edge information that she disseminates to the public with authentic and well-founded spirit. Throughout the decades, it has come to my attention that some of the best physicians that I have worked with and gotten to know come from a background in animal husbandry. Beyond this, Max's love for fitness and exercise affords her a unique vantage point allowing her to establish the fundamental necessity for aerobic and weight-training health.

What I love about this straightforward contribution is that it provides substance along with experiential science. Without fail, if you follow the advice of 'Doc Max', your bones will begin to stand up straight and regain their prominent place in your anatomy. Ironically, even those who eat well can fall into the grips of osteo conditions. There are always two definitive directions I give those suffering from this ever-growing malady. First, you must help the cells press together and solidify, increasing bone density. This is only achieved by an ongoing programme of weightlifting. Next, one must consume a diet that is rich in minerals, not animal based, and, most importantly, uncooked. This prescription has helped thousands of women and even some men remove the shackles of pain and premature aging caused by this potential crippler.

Foreword

Osteoporosis, which was once relegated to a handful of well-off prima donnas, has seemingly become a global plague. Our modern lifestyle that finds us sitting more than moving, and gazing into a screen rather than absorbing nature's vistas, weakens our skeletal structure. Foods high in acidity add a secondary layer to the collapse of your hard tissue. As a young student, I was shocked to watch over a several week period, a human bone disintegrate in a carbonated soda. Our professor surely made his point to the class. Unfortunately, today the majority of us follow a sedentary lifestyle, starving our bodies with the nonsense we consume called 'food'. What a surprise it is for those who are diagnosed with disease. Their first response usually is, 'I live in a healthy way.' People do not acknowledge that over the last several generations, there is a global biology experiment being conducted on humanity. We are the first ever that do not eat from a fresh, nutritious selection. In addition, manual labour (exercise) has been replaced with automation and sedentary work stations. Needless to say, the resulting effect causes a systemic breakdown of the body. 'Use it or lose it' is more than a slogan, it is a fact.

Max Tuck is one of my favourite health educators anywhere on earth. Her strong and vibrant physical persona and keenly sharpened intellect manifest into a perfect example of why we should listen to her. Few follow their passion and walk their talk. This is not the case with Doc Max. Read every word and take it to heart, but most importantly, apply it. If you are concerned about the health of your skeletal structure, there has never been a better manual or blueprint guiding you on how to regain it and maintain it. Thank you so much for presenting the answer to overcoming osteoporosis.

Brian R. Clement

Director, Hippocrates Health Institute, Florida, USA

About the author

I gained my degree in veterinary medicine in 1985 from the Royal Veterinary College, London. As a result of this medical background, I approach all health issues, whether human or animal, from a rigorously scientific perspective. Now a Hippocrates Health Institute-trained health educator as well as a practising vet, I was originally prompted to investigate the importance of nutrition to health by my own collapse with chronic fatigue and Epstein-Barr virus 25 years ago. Since my 'miraculous' recovery, I have run marathons, competed in triathlons, climbed mountains and gained my black belt in karate, in addition to managing my punishing dual-role work schedule. For more information about my other books and services, including the health retreats I run, or to book me as a speaker, please visit me at www.therawfoodscientist.com.

Acknowledgement

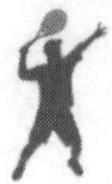

Thanks are due to the many people whose support and input in the creation of this book have been invaluable. To Georgina and the team at Hammersmith Health Books, for seeing the potential; to Alex Burton, my former personal trainer, for his exercise recommendations, and for pushing me beyond what even I believed was possible; to Debbie Pentland for her bone-strengthening exercises and for reminding me why I run; to Rian and Trish for the brainstorming sessions; to Drs Brian and Anna-Maria Clement and the Hippocrates Health Institute team in Florida for the support that they give to thousands of people worldwide.

Special thanks as always go to Stewart Lynch, for his unfailing commitment to my many project ideas, and for his computer expertise, without which I am sure my books and CDs would never have seen the light of day.

Introduction

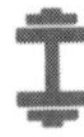

Why do we need another book about osteoporosis? Don't we already know that the disease is just caused by calcium deficiency and lack of exercise? I beg to differ. If it were that simple, we would not be hearing about the disastrous statistics that are outlined in chapter 1, and, for example, the incidence of hip fractures in Canada would not be expected to quadruple by the year 2030.[1] Somehow, the prevention messages (or should that, in some cases, be 'mixed messages'?) are not getting through.

I have a particular interest in bone health. First, because my mother had this diagnosis and I wanted to research how she could reverse the condition. Second, because I have had a fair few broken bones in the past, and I can tell you, it hurts. I don't want anyone else to have to experience the same degree of pain and debility that I have managed to subject myself to in my life. I'm known as a bit of a daredevil, and during my first 18 years on the planet I broke three arms (OK, I broke my right arm twice), my nose, and shattered my coccyx (the base of my spine) – I still have a lump there to this day. Later on I broke two toes in a karate grading when my foot got slammed out of the way by my opponent, and went on to rupture my cruciate ligaments in a skiing accident in which I fell 200 feet on ice. (Alright, so this wasn't a broken bone, but it was actually harder to fix.) I would like to stress at this point that I have very robust bones – it was just that the impact forces in all of these accidents were huge, and more than even my strong frame could withstand. Just imagine what could have happened to someone whose bones were much more fragile.

I do wonder if we would be more inclined to take care of our bones if they were visible. How many skin care products do we see, lining the shelves of every supermarket, pharmacy and specialist store? They give vague promises of 'younger-looking skin' and purport to be 'anti-wrinkle', with the cosmetics industry itself being worth billions a year. We never hear of a 'bone care routine' in the same way in which we hear of a skin care routine (although to make up for this, I have added one at the back of this book, see page 167). What a great pity that is, since the challenges associated with poor bone health far outweigh any physical challenges that one might experience with developing the odd wrinkle or two.

As you progress through this book, you will find that I have not just written it from the perspective of bone health, important though that is. For every element or principle involved in bone care, there are many other whole-body benefits that will be enjoyed as a result.

I am often asked, when I give presentations or conduct private consultations, 'Will a change in diet help with..?'. My answer is always the same. A correctly conducted nutritional regime will improve health at a cellular level, and kick-start the reversal of many disease states, but food alone is not the answer to everything. There are, in my opinion, as many as eight 'Pillars of Health', and an excellent diet is only one of them. The other seven are exercise, rest, sunshine, hydration, stress relief, the cultivation of a positive attitude, and incorporation of some type of spiritual practice or 'life purpose'. These are all as important as each other, and by ignoring one we diminish the benefits of all. We are only as strong as our weakest link.

I have met many people through the years who focused

intently on one of the eight, whilst ignoring all the rest. A friend of mine with whom I did triathlon training in the mid-1990s was incredibly strong and fit, having represented Great Britain at the 1988 Olympics in Seoul. He never fuelled his body correctly for the demands he placed on it, and always laughed at me and my 'rabbit food diet', as he described it. I will always remember going out to dinner with him one night after a particularly heavy circuit training session, and him saying to me, whilst he tucked into a massive plate of spaghetti Bolognese with extra cheese – 'You're too scrawny, lass – you need to eat more lard!' I was never offended by this comment, being proud of my lean, muscular physique, maintained at that time by a high-percentage raw food diet and an intensive exercise programme. A few months later he became unwell with very vague signs that he sadly ignored, believing that because he was fit he was therefore indestructible. He died six months later aged just 34.

Likewise, but in rather sharp contrast to my Olympian friend, I have met numerous people with a very strong religious belief who have ignored the other seven pillars of health, not treating their bodies in the way that I believe their Creator would have wished. I have seen them develop degenerative disease that severely compromised their enjoyment of life, accepting it as 'God's will'. Personally, I don't think people's gods pick on them to suffer. They may just want us to learn something.

So, whilst this book is entitled 'Love Your Bones' and we often think of food as the most important aspect of bone health, you will notice in the following chapters that I have also included some 'non-food' items. If I had not done this, I would be short-changing you, dear reader. Even now, some experts are telling us that osteoporosis is just a deficiency of weight-bearing exercise. But just like the people mentioned above who focused on only one of the eight pillars, I don't want you to focus just on, for example, exercise, or only on the umbrella term 'hormone replacement', in the expectation that it will reverse bone loss.

It may not, for reasons we will come on to. And here I should also mention that whilst scaffolding (i.e. our bone strength) is important, by practising all of the recommendations given here, you may find that other health challenges and minor niggles (or even more major ones) could also be resolved. Brian Clement, Director of the Hippocrates Health Institute in Florida, notices this all the time with guests that present themselves at the Institute for a specific health problem. He hears comments such as 'I came here to recover from cancer, but you didn't tell me that my high blood pressure would also be reversed!', or 'I came here to lose weight, but now I feel more empathy towards my son/daughter/father/mother.'

This is a whole body we live in, my friends. The medical profession may wish to compartmentalise us into different categories according to the sign that presents first, such as cancer, or heart disease, or osteoporosis. Although your main presentation or concern might be osteoporosis, you could be facing additional health challenges, because all of our body systems are related to each other, and lifestyle choices which damage one body system are silently damaging others.

Finally, bear in mind that there are numerous types of 'healthy eating plan', which I will discuss in more detail once we get going. I will give plenty of information on the best type for osteoporosis, and indeed the health of the whole body, as we progress, and in the recipe section at the end of the book. Let's get started, let's get strong, and let's get healthy.

Note: For those who like their scientific references, you will notice that among the research I have cited through the chapters is work that has been performed using animals. This does not mean I agree with this as a method, but given that the research exists it is important to include it here in the sum of our knowledge.

Chapter 1

Some alarming statistics

One of the main reasons I cite for paying attention to bone health throughout our lives is the devastation that bone ill-health can cause over time if we don't. According to the International Osteoporosis Foundation (IOF), the sheer number of people affected is huge:

- Worldwide, osteoporosis causes more than 8.9 million fractures annually, resulting in an osteoporotic fracture every three seconds.[1]
- Osteoporosis is estimated to affect 200 million women worldwide – approximately one-tenth of women aged 60, one-fifth of women aged 70, two-fifths of women aged 80 and two-thirds of women aged 90.[2]
- Osteoporosis affects an estimated 75 million people in Europe, USA and Japan.[3]
- For the year 2000, there were an estimated 9 million new osteoporotic fractures, of which 1.6 million were at the hip, 1.7 million were at the forearm and 1.4 million were clinical vertebral fractures. Europe and the Americas accounted for 51 per cent of all these fractures, while most of the remainder occurred in the Western Pacific region and Southeast Asia.[4]
- Worldwide, one in three women over the age of 50 will experience osteoporotic fractures, as will one in five men aged over 50.[5]

In North America more specifically, according to further data from the IOF, the trends are equally alarming:

- Canada: Osteoporosis affects approximately 1.4 million Canadians, mainly postmenopausal women and the elderly. Osteoporosis affects one in four women and more than one in eight men over the age of 50 years, with one in four men and women having evidence of a vertebral fracture.
- Canada: Almost 30,000 hip fractures occur each year. By the year 2030, the number of hip fractures is expected to quadruple.
- USA: Osteoporosis and low bone mass are currently estimated to be a major public health threat for almost 44 million US women and men aged 50 and older.
- USA: The 44 million people with either osteoporosis or low bone mass represent 55 per cent of the people aged 50 and older in the United States.

Osteoporosis is often referred to as 'the silent killer' because it can be present for many years, often undetected, until a bone suddenly breaks; usually, in women, the hip. A fracture is just the acute manifestation of a chronic long-term problem, and by the time the bone breaks, it can be very difficult to undo the damage. Worryingly, 20 per cent of osteoporotic hip fracture victims die within one year of the fracture occurring, whilst a further 30 per cent are forced into nursing homes. Overall, only 30 per cent of patients manage to recover fully from osteoporotic hip fracture. It therefore follows that to avoid being one of the increasing number of people suffering the devastation that this disease can bring, prevention is the key. However, if you have already been diagnosed, please do not despair, since bone mass can be improved in both sexes, and at any age.

For longevity, wellbeing and reversal of disease states, the dietary regime outlined in the chapters that follow has been demonstrated to give unparalleled results. The correct diet and exercise programme genuinely can rebuild your failing structural elements. It really is time to love your bones and think of them as living, breathing entities, rather than just boring inert scaffolding. They deserve as much attention as your heart, liver, skin and brain. Treat them well and they will support you forever.

Chapter 1 summary

- Osteoporosis is a potentially devastating condition and the worldwide incidence is increasing.
- It is more common in women, but men are not immune from the disease.
- Less than a third of people sustaining an osteoporotic fracture return to a normal life afterwards; a fifth of those who break a hip die within one year.
- Prevention of the disease is key, but osteoporosis can also be reversed with appropriate dietary and lifestyle intervention.

Chapter 2

Bone structure and development: understanding your scaffolding

We often don't give our bones a lot of thought, but there they are, the very essence of our structure, allowing us to enjoy the uninterrupted movement and strength that our daily lives demand. It's often only when we break a bone, or we are given the frightening diagnosis of the life-limiting condition described as osteoporosis, that we might give due consideration to this essential, 'alive' crystalline matrix that lies beneath our muscle mass.

Often considered to be just a boring inert framework that doesn't really do much apart from allow the rest of the bodily structures to be built on and around it, bone is in reality living tissue, with a blood and nerve supply, a highly active internal marrow and an impressive ability to naturally repair itself and restore its own function even after major traumatic injury. In other words, bone tissue is, like many other parts of the body, self-regenerating. Having operated on hundreds of bones during my 30-year career as a surgeon, I can honestly say that the post-operative X-ray follow-up series continues to amaze me, even to this day. Over time, such radiographs show an unmistakable fact: the living tissue regeneration and remodelling is there for all to see. Bone is a fascinating and highly dynamic substance. Once we are aware of this, we can finally appreciate that the elements which allow such tissue restructuring and regeneration have to come from somewhere. That 'somewhere', as true for bone as for any of our other bodily tissues, is our food.

What is bone made of?

Bone is comprised of approximately 35 per cent organic material and 65 per cent mineral-based material. Organic material refers to carbon-based structures, such as proteins. 90 per cent of the organic component of bone is collagen, a structural protein which also gives integrity to the skin, tendons and ligaments. 99 per cent of the mineral-based material is a compound called hydroxyapatite, a crystalline complex of calcium and phosphate. The mineral component provides mechanical rigidity and load-bearing strength to bone, whereas the collagen-based organic matrix provides elasticity and flexibility. Both of these properties are vital to bone's overall strength and resistance to fracture. Bone tissue is the body's largest store of minerals, and as such is closely involved in mechanisms that regulate the body's acid/alkali balance, which you'll learn more about in chapter 4. The formation and maintenance of bone are under the control of numerous cells, hormones and growth factors which are discussed in more detail below, and in the chapters that follow.

Anatomically, bone has two major components: cortical bone, which is solid, dense and surrounds the bone marrow, and trabecular bone, which is a honeycomb-like network of plates and rods in the bone marrow compartment in the centre.

Bone cells

There are three major cellular components to bone, which are:

Osteoblasts – the bone-building cells
Osteocytes – osteoblasts that have become incorporated into the bone matrix

Osteoclasts – cells that remove worn-out bone.

All three types of cell are essential to the correct functioning and strength of the bones. Let's look at them all in a little more detail.

Osteoblasts

Osteoblasts secrete the organic matrix of collagen and other structural proteins, such as osteocalcin and osteopontin, in a dense array of cross-linked 'ropes' that give bone a very high tensile strength; see also 'bone glue' below. The osteoblasts also secrete the minerals from which the crystalline hydroxyapatite compound is formed: the inorganic mineral component of bone which gives it its rigidity.

Osteocalcin is a protein which deserves special mention, since it is closely involved in ensuring that the hydroxyapatite crystalline structure forms the correct shape for greatest strength and rigidity. The formation of the osteocalcin protein involves two important steps, fascinating to those interested in organic chemistry, which involve vitamin D and vitamin K2; both of which you will read more about in chapter 9. When osteocalcin comes into contact with calcium ions, the protein folds in a special way to allow it to 'dock' onto the hydroxyapatite crystal, and add more calcium where it is needed, allowing the bone to grow. In organised groups of connected cells, osteoblasts deposit minerals into the organic matrix, subsequently forming a very strong and dense mineralised tissue known as the mineralised matrix.

Osteocytes

These cells are former osteoblasts that have, in effect, become buried in the bone matrix. They possess long dendrites: thin, finger-like processes that protrude from the cell surface and sense the forces which are applied to the bone. They are the 'communicators' within the bone structure, and signal to the other bone cells whether to make more bone, or reduce further bone development. They perform a very important function during exercise: when the bones are loaded and under stress from muscle and tendon tension, osteocytes convey these messages to the osteoblasts and initiate bone strengthening and further development as a response to these forces.

Recent studies have also indicated that depriving the osteocytes of oxygen is a factor in the determination of overall bone strength.[1] Less oxygen means reduced strength of bone as a result of lack of stimulation of the bone-building mechanism. It is possible therefore (although more research is needed) that anything which delivers higher levels of oxygen to the tissues might have a positive effect on bone health. Exercise is just one way by which tissues become more highly oxygenated; others depend on our food and lifestyle choices.

Osteoclasts

Osteoclasts are the cells which break down old, worn-out bone. They too are under the control of hormones and other chemical regulators. Osteoclasts perform numerous important functions, including ensuring that the bones do not overgrow, preventing them from becoming too thick or dense. They are also involved in remodelling of the bone so that it retains its correct shape, for example during fracture healing when bone calluses are remodelled. In post-menopausal women, the activity of osteoclasts is often greater than that of osteoblasts, resulting in a decline in bone mineral density and net bone loss as time goes on. As a result, osteoclasts are considered by some to be the 'bad guys', but this is not necessarily correct. Many drug interventions for osteoporosis focus on blocking osteoclast activity; you'll read more about this, and its potential side effects, in chapter 10.

Chapter 2

'Bone glue'

Discovered by Professor Paul Hansma, with publication of the discovery in the journal *Nature* in 2005, 'bone glue' could be the missing link in our knowledge of how our bones work to resist fracture. Inspired by some very interesting mechanical properties of abalone shell, which is 97 per cent crystalline calcium carbonate and 3 per cent organic material, Professor Hansma initially wanted to investigate why it was that the incorporation of just 3 per cent organic material in the shell made it 3000 times more resistant to fracture than 100 per cent pure crystalline calcium carbonate. Could such a small proportion of organic material really make that amount of difference? And if so, how? It turns out that it does.

Professor Hansma not only ascertained how this is possible on a molecular level (you can read about some of the science, which I find fascinating, on page 10), but subsequently investigated to see if this incredible property of abalone shell existed elsewhere in nature. Fortunately for us, it does – in our bones. Essentially, bone glue amounts to a physical phenomenon which is measured by an atomic force microscope. This breakthrough science is leading on to the development of exciting technology for the more accurate evaluation of fracture risk and earlier detection of people at risk of fractures; something that you can read more about on pages 15–17.

I was very fortunate, just prior to going to print, to be able to ask Professor Hansma some questions about bone glue, which will aid in our understanding of how bones work and what determines their strength. This is quite scientific, so if you're not scientifically minded you're allowed to skip this section; neither of us will be offended.

A short scientific interview with Professor Hansma

Max Tuck (MT): What is bone glue? We know apparently that it is not collagen, but do you have more information about what exactly it is?

Paul Hansma (PH): The current best evidence[2, 3] is that heavily phosphorylated proteins such as osteopontin and bone sialoprotein are primary constituents of bone glue. In the presence of calcium ions, strong ionic bonds are formed between phosphate groups on the same phosphorylated protein polymer or between phosphorylated polymers. It is important to know that proteins like osteopontin and bone sialoprotein are known to have no tertiary structure. That is, they do not fold into compact structures of the sort biology books are full of. Rather they remain as unstructured, unfolded polymers, which are ideal for their putative role as adhesives.

MT: Can bone glue regenerate?

PH: Yes! The osteocytes that are maintained by the body at high density and correspondingly high metabolic 'cost' can produce and secrete these proteins. My own theory is that one of the major roles of the osteocytes is to replenish degenerated bone glue. In support of this theory is the fact that osteocytes are known to produce more of these proteins in the presence of shear stress of fluid moving over the cells, which occurs when bone is strained – the strains create fluid flow in the canaliculi that contain the processes of the osteocytes. This could be an elegant mechanism. Too much strain in a bone results in the production of bone glue to reinforce it.

MT: Is bone glue evenly distributed through the skeletal structure or is it more concentrated in certain parts of the body?

PH: It is more concentrated where it is needed, for example at the cement lines in bone, which are regions of weakness because they have no mineralised collagen fibrils crossing the lines to reinforce them. Osteopontin is also, unfortunately, present in gluing plaque to the insides of arteries! [See also chapter 7.] Phosphorylated proteins are such good glues that the body is very careful about where they occur. One of the routine blood tests most people get is for their Alkaline Phosphatase level. This is an enzyme with the job of dephosphorylating proteins in the blood to prevent things sticking together.

MT: The sacrificial bonds, which you explain and so clearly demonstrate in your lectures and videos; is there anything that potentially stops them from reforming, thereby affecting fracture resistance?

PH: Absence of water will keep them from reforming, so good hydration is essential. This is one reason that mechanical tests on damp bone (or, even worse, dry bone) are so different from tests on bone that is in solution, like it is in the body. This is one reason that tests with the Osteoprobe [see below] are so valuable: they test the bone inside a patient's body, where it is in its natural environment.

MT: Do we know how the bone glue gets into the bones in the first place? Does it form in the foetus, and which tissue produces it?

PH: A lot is known about the production of proteins, including osteopontin and bone sialoprotein during development. In fact, in the past it was believed that their only role was in development for promoting or inhibiting mineralisation at appropriate times. The idea that these proteins have a mechanical role is relatively new and slowly gaining acceptance.

It's not just bone cells

Anything that affects the cells involved in bone building and remodelling will in turn affect not only bone strength, but many other physiological processes throughout the body, since cell receptors that are present in bone are also found in numerous other tissues. Whilst it is very important to look after our bones as we age, it doesn't stop there. The good news is that anything that is beneficial to bone health will also positively affect our health in other ways. Indeed, the dietary regimes and lifestyle choices that promote our bone health and strength will have the 'side effect' of reducing the susceptibility to cancer, heart disease, diabetes, stroke, obesity and many other common diseases. You'll find out more about these added benefits as we progress through the chapters.

How can we measure bone strength?

'The best way to test the strength of a bone is to break it.' These are the words of Professor Hansma, and in effect, he is absolutely right. Ideally, to work out our risk of fracture, we need to take a bone out of the body, hit it with a hammer and see how much force is required to smash it to bits. Fortunately, modern-day research is not this brutal, but when we consider how to detect if we are at risk of fracturing a bone following, for example, a simple fall, we need to look at ways of measuring the strength and resilience of our bones to such trauma. Current methods are not 100 per cent accurate in this determination, since bone density is only part of the equation, as you'll see from the diagram below.

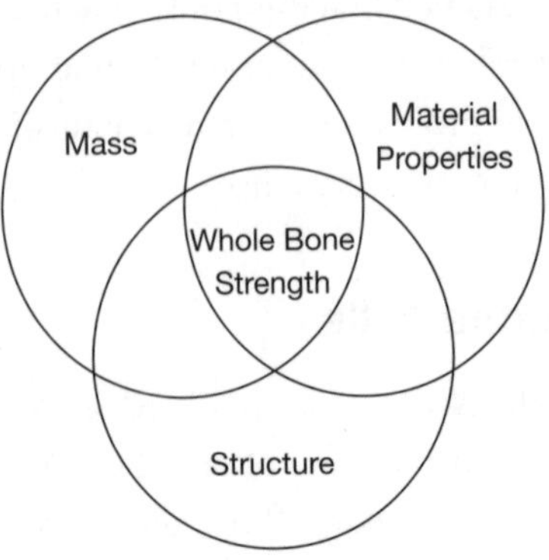

Image provided courtesy of ActiveLife Scientific Inc, manufacturers of OsteoProbe and BioDent technologies, Santa Barbara California, USA.

Chapter 2

Current methods for evaluating bone health

DEXA (DXA) scanning

We often hear about bone density measurement, but the density of the bone is not always an accurate indication of how likely it is to break when an external force is applied to it. Bone density is measured by a dual-energy X-ray absorptiometry (DEXA or DXA) scan, which is an assessment of how much calcium is present in the bone. (Read more about calcium in chapters 3 and 7.) The scan is essentially a two-dimensional X-ray, which provides an estimate of the mineral density of the bone in the region studied. Common areas to examine are the total hip, femoral neck, spine and wrist. Since the test is based on two-dimensional imaging, and of course bones are three-dimensional, it gives an estimate of density rather than a direct measurement.

The accuracy of this density estimate is affected by many factors. Smaller people with smaller bones, (i.e. those with a small frame and low body weight, such as myself) will achieve lower scores, machines from different manufacturers might give non-comparable results, different anatomical sites might give different results for men but not women, and any abnormalities in the area being scanned, such as surgery or compression fractures, will also affect the results. The density measurement is generally reported as a 'T-score', which is the amount of deviation from the average reading seen in a young adult of the same sex. The reading you get from a DEXA scan is therefore not an absolute value, but one that is compared to general population statistics.

Despite these limitations, DEXA scans can provide some useful information about bone health. While the T-score cannot tell an individual their absolute risk of fracture, it does give an estimate of relative risk, the risk compared to others with 'normal' density. It is currently regarded, in the medical profession, as the best measurement test available to provide this information.

However, it is still stated that a DEXA scan cannot diagnose over 80 per cent of the 200 million people worldwide who may be at risk from a fracture.[4]

The DEXA scan tells us about the amount of bone (the quantity), but not the quality of the bone itself. And quality, the underlying strength of the bone material, is probably the most important consideration. As with any structural material, both the quantity of that substance and its underlying quality are critical in determining its overall strength.

Is there a better way?

New techniques are currently being examined to evaluate whether they are better predictors of fracture risk than bone mineral density (BMD) measurements via DEXA scans. As we now know, DEXA scans do not give information regarding the health and thickness of cortical and trabecular bone, only the overall density, which, as we have seen, does not always accurately correlate with the likelihood of a fracture and the resistance to applied forces. Greater accuracy may be provided via CT scanning, which gives an indication of bone structure, and such techniques are being used experimentally in Europe to evaluate better ways of predicting fracture risk.[5] The disadvantage of this method, aside from cost, so far has been that a relatively high dose of radiation is required, although early results are encouraging.

Results from recent studies using new applications of ultrasound techniques and MRI imaging are becoming available, and preliminary studies show the value of these new techniques in the measurement of bone structure, to estimate bone strength and assess fracture risk more accurately. However, to become clinically useful, many of these methods require further investigation to increase their ease of use and decrease their cost. They are techniques which might show us, in the future, that we were possibly worrying unduly about a low BMD reading, and that it was not necessarily giving us the full picture on our fracture risk.

The FRAX Algorithm

The FRAX Algorithm has been developed by the World Health Organisation (WHO) to give an indication of 10-year hip or other major osteoporotic fracture risk.[6] It is based on individual patient models and integrates clinical risk factors with BMD (bone mineral density) measured at the hip. Where BMD readings are not available, charts have been produced that can be used with body mass index (BMI) readings, which is calculated by taking your weight in kg and dividing it by your height in metres squared. As an example, I weigh 53 kg and I am 1.65 metres tall. To calculate my BMI, I multiply 1.65 by 1.65. This gives 2.72. I then divide my weight (53 kg) by 2.72, giving me a BMI of 19.48.

Risk factors listed in the questionnaire are quite limited. They include smoking, previous osteoporotic fracture, a parent sustaining a hip fracture, use of glucocorticoid (steroid) drugs, consumption of more than three units of alcohol per day (see chapters 4 and 10), and being affected by rheumatoid arthritis or secondary osteoporosis. It does not take into consideration any of the other factors that you will discover, through this book, to be detrimental to bone strength; for example high animal protein consumption (chapter 5) and a sedentary lifestyle (chapter 12) to name but two. It is a useful tool nonetheless for those who do not have access to other diagnostic modalities.

A long-awaited breakthrough

Some very good news on bone quality testing is just now emerging from the USA, and a new 'bone probe', invented by Professor Hansma, has been developed by a company called ActiveLife

Scientific in California. They have so far developed two types of bone probe: the OsteoProbe, which is currently being used for research purposes only, and the BioDent probe, which has been the subject of numerous published studies. 'Microindentation', which is measured with these probes, could indeed be the new buzzword in the diagnosis of osteoporosis, and in the future may become the gold standard for assessment of fracture risk, if the early, encouraging studies prove to be correct.[7, 8] By using bone probes, it has been ascertained, so far, that diminished bone quality in the tibia (shin bone) is a good indicator of the quality of bone throughout the body.

Briefly, microindentation is a technique of using a microscopic probe, inserted into the bone, to give a reference reading of how hard the bone tissue is; i.e. how resistant it is to insertion of the probe. Previous attempts at measuring such forces have been difficult, since when you push on something, be it bone or anything else, it moves away from you. Professor Hansma's device uses the concept of 'reference point indentation (RPI)' which gets around this problem. The readings obtained relate to how easy, in effect, it is to insert the probe into the bone: the greater the resistance to insertion, the stronger the bone, and vice versa. The wonderful science behind this instrument is as follows (from Professor Hansma's website):

> *The Reference Point Indentation instrument will measure microscopic materials properties of the bones of living patients with accuracy and ease. Our hypothesis is, and our preliminary results are in agreement, that a measure of microscopic fracture resistance with the Reference Point Indentation instrument in an individual's bone correlates with their resistance to macroscopic bone fractures, or, stated another way, their overall bone fracture risk. Indentation testing is already well-established as a powerful tool in characterizing mechanical properties of materials.*

> *Fundamental research has revealed that bone fractures begin when the organic matrix of the bone, or 'glue' holding mineralized collagen fibrils together, fails causing crack propagation. Preliminary results with the Reference Point Indentation instrument have shown that an individual's susceptibility to this fundamental failure mode can be measured by indentation tests in which bone is forced, on a microscopic scale, into the same types of failure – separation of mineralized collagen fibrils – that is the root event of bone fractures. Preliminary results with the Reference Point Indentation instrument have also shown that the necessary measurement can be performed on bone that is still covered with soft tissue (skin).*

The great news for the future of our diagnosis system is that the probe is small and easy to use; small enough to be stored on a doctor's desktop, and, as such, has great potential to become incorporated into general use. I, for one, would be very happy to undergo a test such as this; it eliminates the need for exposure to ionizing radiation (X-rays and CT scans) and takes very little time. It could well become the future of accurate diagnostics and fracture risk assessment.

Chapter 2 summary

- Bone is made up of organic (protein) and inorganic (mineral) components.
- There are three types of active cells in the bone: those which build bone, those which break it down, and those which act as communicators.
- 'Bone glue' is a fascinating new discovery which could, in the future, give us an amazing insight into bone health and strength.
- DEXA scans have their limitations and might not be the best way in which to diagnose patients who are most at

risk of fractures. Recent developments in technology, such as the OsteoProbe, could pave the way for better diagnosis and earlier detection in the future.

Chapter 3

I'm already weaned, thanks!

Have you ever stopped to wonder why it is that humans appear to be the only mammal that insists on drinking milk after weaning age? Ever since I began studying the biological sciences in high school, this odd phenomenon has always perplexed me. I perhaps had a greater interest in the habit of dairy product consumption than most. My childhood eczema was a direct result of consuming pasteurised cow's milk, so I eliminated all dairy products from my diet at the age of 15. I am still stunned, to this day, that intelligent people continue to ask me questions about my bone density and where I get my calcium from, having been dairy-free for over 35 years. And likewise, the people who assume that I therefore use soya milk instead. Why is it that the consumption of cooked milk, from the wrong species of mammal, past weaning age is considered to be a natural, and even beneficial thing for the adult human to do? Sadly, from the research that I have conducted, it appears to come down to two major factors: brainwashing and indoctrination.

Is the dairy industry in control of our bone health?

The dairy industry pays governments worldwide a large amount of money to promote the use of its products. I noticed this at first hand when I went to have a bone scan, aged 40. I sat in a depressing waiting room, with several elderly ladies who were exhibiting very severe signs of osteoporosis, waiting for my scan. One thing that struck me immediately was the choice of posters on the walls. 'Drink milk for strong bones,' said one. 'Milk, have you got it?' reiterated another. And at the bottom of each poster, in almost imperceptibly small print, was stated: 'Information provided by the Milk Marketing Board' (now rebranded as The Dairy Council). Well, what a surprise – a vested interest.

Brendan Brazier, the Canadian Ironman Triathlete, and author of *The Thrive Diet* and *Thrive Fitness*, states that the dairy industry pulled off an almost impossible feat just over 100 years ago. He relates that dairy products, at the beginning of the 20th century, were not listed as a food group. As a result of the rapid changes in the industry and a move to larger commercial organisation of dairy farming, particularly in North America, the lobbying powers of the industry enabled dairy products to be added to the early 'food pyramid' as an accepted food group. This was a triumph for marketing and lobbying and has had a massive impact on our observed health, or demise of it, in the Western world over the past 100 years.

You can tell what's coming next, can't you? I am going to tell you that for protection of bone strength, and prevention and reversal of osteoporosis, one of the most essential things you must do is eliminate all dairy products from your diet. For those who are sceptical still that the adult human can survive, nay thrive, without the incorporation of the mammary secretions of a large ruminant into their diet, I would ask this: does milk (whether from the correct species of mammal or not, pasteurised or otherwise) contain any element that cannot be obtained from a different source in the plant kingdom? I am yet to find one.

For all my vegan readers, you may be wondering why I have included a discussion on dairy products in this book – of course, you are already following a plant-based diet and therefore may consider this tip to be irrelevant. The reason, to me, is clear. I want to ensure that I leave no stone unturned in my recommendations and to highlight why the consumption of dairy products does nothing positive for bone density. You can then pass this information on to others who may be in need of it. False information is so deeply ingrained in our society that we sometimes need to have a very strong counter-argument to reinforce our own belief system. I think it's time for some science.

The link between dairy consumption and osteoporosis

Which nations in the world have the highest incidence of osteoporosis? Which nations are the world's highest consumers of dairy products? If we are supposed to be using milk and its derivatives for strong bones, why it is that the good people of these nations who are behaving in the way that the dairy lobby wants them to, are rewarded with weak, brittle bones and fractures? Look at the evidence. Now we could say that there are 'lies, damned lies, and statistics', and it is true that statistics can be manipulated in such a way that they can be made to tell us practically anything. But in this particular instance, the evidence appears to be very clear. Dairy product consumption seems to be positively associated with hip fractures when studying trends in large population groups.[1] Why would this be?

Interestingly, whilst the bones of women in the countries with the highest dairy product consumption may seem, on average, to be denser than those with low dairy consumption, this does not appear to protect them from fractures.[2]

Bone density, whilst relatively easy to measure with a DEXA scan, appears to be only part of the picture. When we look more closely at such studies, some interesting findings present themselves, notably that those with higher BMD (bone mineral density) on DEXA scans seem more likely to be prone to hip fracture. This odd statistic certainly requires clarification, and indicates that a higher BMD is not necessarily the key to bone health. What seems to be much more important is the quality of bone, which is not something that a DEXA scan can easily evaluate, since it only gives an indication of calcium content. I go deeper into this apparent paradox in chapter 7, in which I discuss calcium in more detail; as mentioned in chapter 2, other methods of evaluating bone resilience are being developed which could be of considerably greater value than DEXA scans.

Baby food

Let's get back to the consideration that health-conscious people should, in my opinion, be avoiding dairy products; not just for reasons of bone health, but also for the avoidance of other disease processes discussed at the end of this chapter. Firstly, there is the issue that milk is a baby food. Yes, that's right: you're already weaned, you don't need it. But one of the main problems with it is the way in which we consume it as adult humans. We choose the pasteurised products of the cow, a very large mammal whose high-protein, high-fat milk is designed to allow its calf to gain 400 pounds in weight in its first year of life. As a slight digression, I was amused to hear in February 2011 that a restaurant in London had just started serving ice cream made from human breast milk. People were calling in to the local radio station saying how disgusting that was and questioning why anyone in their right mind would want to order it. I had to laugh. They didn't consider that a food specifically designed for them when they were babies was appropriate to make ice cream from, but were quite happy to accept it from a cow. It was a sad indication of how warped we, as a society, seem to have become.

Digressions aside, by cooking the milk prior to consumption we alter how we utilise it. The calcium[3] and possibly other bone-strengthening minerals we need are less bioavailable. It has been speculated that this is the case because the heating process destroys the enzyme that would allow those minerals to be incorporated into our structure. Additionally, and we will cover this in more depth in later chapters, pasteurised dairy products are a high-protein, high-acid residue food. When we consume products that leave an acidic residue, and there are others besides pasteurised dairy, we need to rebalance the acidity with alkaline minerals, coming from the body's largest alkaline mineral resource – the bones.

According to David Wolfe, the respected researcher on all aspects of longevity in relation to living foods, humans have the ability to digest and assimilate the minerals in unpasteurised dairy products up until about the age of 15. Thereafter this ability starts to wane, disappearing entirely within approximately two years. This ability may also be influenced by the fact that for calcium to be assimilated into the bones, we need good levels of magnesium. Magnesium is discussed more fully in a later chapter, but the calcium to magnesium ratio is critical for calcium to be utilised for laying down new bone. An unfavourable ratio causes calcium to be moved out of the bones and deposited in the tissues. Dairy products are too low in magnesium ever to be useful in bone building.

Too much protein

We will come on to talk about protein and its damaging effects on bone health later (see chapter 4), but standard dairy products, whether pasteurised or otherwise, are a high-fat, high-protein food. They are designed for a period of time when the infant is growing at its most rapid rate. If we needed another reason to question their appropriateness, here it is: human breast milk, designed to nourish an infant through its most rapid growth stage, is approximately 1.5 per cent protein, with a higher fat content than cow's milk, to allow for rapid development of the human brain and nerves. Cow's milk protein content ranges from 3.5 to 4 per cent. If we only need 1.5 per cent protein at our life stage of most rapid growth, why is a product containing twice the amount of protein considered to be even remotely appropriate? As adults, we have stopped growing and no longer need this high level of fat and protein. When it comes to protein, more is definitely not better. Many studies have shown the detrimental effect of high-protein diets on bone density, which will be discussed later.

Before leaving the protein story, it is worth mentioning that the type of protein in cow's milk is not the same as that in human milk. The proteins in milk can be divided into two categories: caseins and whey proteins. Human milk contains these in a ratio of 40:60 respectively; while in cow's milk the ratio of casein to whey proteins is 80:20. Since we now know that the amount of total protein in cow's milk is more than double that of human milk, cow's milk clearly contains considerably more casein than human milk. Casein can be difficult to digest; interestingly it is used to make certain types of glue, which is not generally a product that would be deemed fit for human consumption. Casein has been linked to a range of diseases and allergies, including type 1 diabetes (see below).

What, therefore, about children? We have discussed that adults do not need dairy products, but could we potentially be causing harm to the bone development of children by eliminating dairy product consumption? Not according to the authors of a study published in the journal *Pediatrics* in 2005. Following extensive review of the evidence, the authors concluded that 'Scant evidence supports nutrition guidelines focused specifically on increasing milk or other dairy product intake for promoting child and adolescent bone mineralization.'[4]

Ultimately, pasteurised dairy products therefore seem to give us a triple whammy in favour of bone degeneration – high protein, high acid residue and lack of assimilation of the very minerals that we were hoping to find in the products themselves. They should be given a very wide berth indeed.

Other health challenges associated with dairy product consumption

The consumption of dairy products does more than just damage the health of our bones, despite what the dairy industry would love us to believe. Let's look at some other challenges we might face over the years that are linked to drinking milk and eating butter, cheese and yogurt.

Allergies

My years of childhood suffering with eczema and endless steroid creams (which did nothing to solve the problem) were a direct result of dairy consumption: I am allergic to casein, one of the milk proteins mentioned above. Additionally, a large proportion of the world's population is lactose-intolerant. Lactose is a milk sugar, and lactose intolerance is generally associated with digestive disturbances such as bloating, gas and potentially more severe problems such as Crohn's disease. But if you are also looking to enhance the appearance and health of your skin, eliminating dairy products is a great place to start. There are more skin health tips to be found in my book *The Whole Body Solution*, also published by Hammersmith Health Books.

Asthma

Many naturopathic doctors have been able to treat asthma in their patients just by getting them to eliminate dairy products. Improvements are often seen within as little as two weeks. The debate as to whether dairy products really do generate increased mucus formation in the body will no doubt continue, but if your respiratory system needs extra help, eliminating milk and cheese could well be just what it needs.

Cancer

One of the main causative factors for the development of breast cancer is known to be lifetime cumulative exposure to oestrogen, and approximately 80 per cent of all exogenous (environmental) oestrogen derives from the consumption of dairy products.[5] Insulin-like Growth Factor-1 (IGF-1) is a compound which, under unhealthy conditions, promotes malignancy, metastasis and cell division, and it also interferes with cellular apoptosis (programmed cell death). The body makes small quantities of this hormone as required for its biological functions, but additionally it is present in dairy products and is considered to be one of the ways in which dairy product consumption stimulates the cancer process; particularly in relation to prostate cancer.[6] Prostate cancer is now affecting one in six men in North America, and those who consume the most dairy products have twice the incidence of the disease, with four times the metastasis rate, compared with those whose consumption is minimal.

Cardiovascular disease

Whilst we know that cholesterol is not the whole story in relation to cardiovascular disease risk, it remains one of the biomarkers for its assessment. Dairy products contribute significant levels of fat and cholesterol to the diet, and are the number one source of dietary saturated fat in North America. The long-running Adventists Study in the USA indicates that fatal cardiovascular disease is twice as likely in those who consume dairy products as those who do not.[7]

Diabetes

Type 1 (juvenile onset) diabetes is a devastating condition which involves the destruction of the beta (insulin-producing) cells of the pancreas in children. Without endogenous insulin, blood sugar levels cannot be controlled without frequent injections of insulin, derived from the pancreas of a pig. It is well documented that a protein present in cow's milk can trigger the onset of type-1 diabetes,[8] but despite this, and the fact that the incidence of type 1 diabetes is 36 times more common in Finland (high dairy consumption) than it is in Japan (low dairy consumption), the dairy lobby insists that milk is an essential component of a child's diet. I, and numerous health experts and researchers far more qualified than I am, beg to differ.

Multiple sclerosis and other degenerative diseases

MS (multiple sclerosis), and other neurodegenerative diseases such as Parkinson's disease, seem to be more prevalent in populations with high dairy product consumption. In the case of Parkinson's, people with the greatest dairy product intake have twice the incidence of the disease of those with a more moderate consumption. The main culprit is suspected to be neurodegenerative chemicals that concentrate in the milk. Such chemicals are not inactivated by pasteurisation. Proponents of dairy product consumption might argue that these chemicals could be avoided by using organic milk. This could well be the case, but organic dairy products still contain exactly the same high-fat, high-protein and high-IGF-1 triggering levels as their non-organic counterparts, so in my opinion this is not an adequate solution. In the case of MS, it is notable that the incidence of the disease increases the further away from the equator that you live. MS is discussed in greater detail in relation to vitamin D in chapter 9.

Rheumatoid arthritis

An aggressive, autoimmune-linked form of arthritis, rheumatoid arthritis can occur in people of all ages, causing significant loss of mobility. Dairy products have been identified in numerous population studies to be a trigger factor for the increase of pain and inflammation in the joints of sufferers, and eliminating them often brings considerable relief. Adopting a low-fat vegan diet has been demonstrated to be beneficial to people affected by this disease.[9]

Chapter 3 summary

- Dairy products are a poor source of calcium and do not contribute to bone health and strength.
- Nations with the highest dairy product consumption have the highest prevalence of osteoporosis and fractures.
- Dairy products are relatively low in magnesium, a vital mineral for bone health.
- Dairy product consumption can lead to a host of other health challenges, including, but not restricted to, cancer, cardiovascular disease, type 1 diabetes and MS.

Chapter 4

Acidity – your worst enemy

Acid / alkali, or pH, balance is something we are starting to hear a lot about in natural health circles; indeed, some best-selling health books have focused on this very topic. Many people are still unfortunately under the erroneous assumption that all unprocessed food is good because it is all alkaline and therefore it doesn't matter what you eat as long as it is a 'wholefood'. Sorry, but this assumption is not true. Initially we need to have a look at a bit of chemistry to really understand what's going on with this talk of acid and alkali balance.

pH is a scale of measurement of the acidity or alkalinity of any given substance. It runs from pH 1 (as acidic as you can get) to pH 14 (as alkaline as you can get). I always wanted to know, in early school chemistry classes, why it was called pH, especially with a small p and a capital H. I was pedantic like that. For anyone else of the same disposition, the 'p' stands for 'concentration of' (from Latin) and the H stands for the Hydrogen atom. That's it, nothing more spectacular than that. But the pH scale and how our food fits into it is one of the most vital things we need to know about, particularly when it relates to rebuilding our bone structure.

All food, after it has been metabolised, leaves a residue in our tissues that is either on the acid side or on the alkaline side of the scale. A few things are right in the centre at pH 7 (neutral), such as most types of water (but see also below). The reason our pH balance is so critical is because of our absolute human necessity to keep our blood at pH 7.365 (slightly alkaline). If it deviates even slightly towards acidic, such as in the life-threatening condition of metabolic acidosis, our red blood cells go into a group hug and it's all over. For this reason, blood pH hardly changes, ever. Some individual cells in the body are much more forgiving than the blood, and cellular pH can drop as low as 3.4 before those cells die, but they will almost certainly have become highly dysfunctional long before that.

We have a precisely controlled homeostatic mechanism to ensure that the blood always remains within its tightly specified pH range, and this involves movement of alkaline elements into the blood if pH drops even slightly too low, and acidic elements if it goes too high. This is simple, and very effective. However, these acidic and alkaline elements need to come from somewhere, and the two main minerals used to counteract low pH (acidity) are calcium and magnesium. Where is the body's largest supply of these minerals? You guessed it – the bones; your scaffolding.[1] The kidneys are also involved in this mechanism, leading some sceptics to state that it doesn't matter what you eat because it will not alter the pH of your blood. As we progress through this chapter, you will find out that the foods with the more alkaline pH are the very same foods which contain many of the nutrients that we need for good bone health. I'd like to point out that this is probably not a coincidence.

What contributes to acidity?

Life in general tends to push our bodies more towards greater acidity. Metabolic by-products tend to be acidic. Air pollution, particularly if there is a high concentration of carbon dioxide in the air, makes us more acidic (carbon dioxide is an acidic molecule). Some authors have even postulated that acid rain might make us more prone to osteoporosis.[2] Exercise, vital for our health and wellbeing, creates tissue acidity. Stress and over secretion of adrenaline lower the bodily pH. Smoking, in addition to all of its other negative effects on health, causes increased tissue acidity, largely due to the inhalation of highly toxic carbon monoxide. Smoking is a very strong correlator for osteoporosis,[3] as is high caffeine consumption, and caffeine is an acid-forming molecule. Alcohol consumption also leads to a lower than ideal bodily pH.

Prescription medications, in particular non-steroidal anti-inflammatory drugs, are acidic in nature. Even negative thoughts and emotions can leave an acidic residue, shown by the fascinating emerging science of psychoneuroimmunology. We therefore need to ensure that most of the food we eat on a daily basis leaves an alkaline residue to counterbalance these potentially adverse effects. Alkaline residue foods give us alkaline minerals which are essential to incorporate into the bone matrix. Acid forming foods need to be minimised and in some cases eliminated altogether for a period of time to allow the bones a chance to regenerate, and many studies indicate that metabolic acidic load is one of the prime causes of reduced bone mineralisation.[4]

Let's look at the best alkalising foods, and the worst acidic offenders that must be eliminated for bone rebuilding. Firstly, the 'good guys'.

The 'good guys'

Green leaves

It's interesting to note that every part of a plant has a slightly different pH. At the top, the leaves are always alkaline. Stems of plants tend to have a more neutral pH, and lower still, the roots are more acidic. So in my opinion, and in that of many leading health experts, green leaves should make up the bulk of one's diet. They are usually highly mineralised, rich in chlorophyll and alkaline elements and an excellent source of bone-building substances. It is even quoted by mainstream nutritionists that kale and broccoli contain considerably more bioavailable calcium than milk. Now we already know from chapter 3 that milk is useless as a source of bioavailable calcium, but this is mainstream nutrition speaking, so for them to admit it is really quite something. We have considerable evidence that increasing the intake of greens is the key to addressing many modern-day health challenges, and the great thing here is that there is absolutely nothing controversial about greens! Now of course within the various health circles there are greens, greens and still more greens, so a little additional clarification is required.

Wheatgrass juice (a daily 2-oz shot) is at the top of my list for daily intake of greens for the prevention and reversal of osteoporosis. Some of the most successful mammals on the planet are the large herbivores. What do they eat to grow their big strong muscular bodies, which in turn are supported by strongly mineralised bones? Grass, and more grass, with a few herbs and weeds thrown in, obtained from the fields and grasslands they graze on. Now humans, of course, are not natural grass eaters. This is obvious because otherwise there would not be the observed demand for electric lawnmowers.

As a result of its structure, and high cellulose content, we cannot access the elements in wheatgrass without first juicing it; we possess neither the teeth nor the digestive structure to break down cellulose. But when we do juice wheatgrass, we take in anything up to 92 minerals, depending on how the wheatgrass is grown. Humans have an absolute biological need for 60 minerals, and can assimilate a total of 92 when they are present in food. Wheatgrass juice contains a predominance of alkaline minerals and is one of the absolute staples for improvement of bone mineralisation over time.

Seaweeds are also an excellent source of alkaline minerals.

It was Jacques Cousteau who famously told us that the future of nutrition was to be found in the sea, and I don't believe he was talking about eating fish. A regular intake of sea vegetables provides additional alkaline minerals as well as iodine, which feeds the thyroid gland and therefore plays an important part in regulation of the metabolism.

Organic salad leaves are next on the list. Choose from an extensive list including collard greens, rocket (arugula), kale, parsley, bok choi, watercress... the list is almost inexhaustible. Spinach deserves a special mention here. It does contain a good spectrum of alkaline minerals but they are not as bioavailable as we would ideally like due to the presence of oxalates in their structure, which tend to bind the calcium. Spinach does however contain useful minerals that have other benefits, so it should therefore not be disregarded.

Sprouted green foods, such as alfalfa sprouts, broccoli sprouts, red clover and radish sprouts, are also highly alkalising, as are sunflower greens and pea shoots. They can be consumed in abundance for their beneficial properties, particularly when incorporated into juices. Sprouted food is also a fantastic addition to the diet for whole-body benefits, and many phytonutrients are concentrated in the sprouted foods. For example, broccoli sprouts have up to 50 times the concentration of sulforaphane, a type of isothiocyanate (a potent anti-cancer nutrient), than the mature broccoli plant.

Liquid blue-green algae are a popular food supplement and also very alkalising, with a pH of 9. We can't base our whole diet on algae, but for an extra boost of chlorophyll and alkalinity they can be very beneficial. Liquid blue-green algae can be added to your daily green juice, and has many benefits as a result of its protein content, and spectrum of essential healthy fats.

Vegetables

Many vegetables are also on the alkaline side of neutral, but not quite as alkaline-forming as the green leaves. Raw organic garden vegetables can be eaten in abundance in salads and contain many beneficial elements for bone strength. It is interesting to note that some of the most alkaline-forming raw vegetables can become the most acidic when cooked, such as potatoes and tomatoes. Ripe raw tomatoes are a very alkalising fruit, and raw potato juice is something that has been used as a natural treatment for arthritis in Swedish health clinics for many years. However, cooked tomatoes and potatoes leave a very acidic residue in the body, which is a good reason to avoid cooked starchy vegetables when wanting to re-establish a more correct pH balance. Since the standard Western diet tends to incorporate a lot of potatoes, we really need a re-think of our 'traditional' diet in my opinion, and substitution of potatoes by other less harmful starchy vegetables would be a beneficial starting point. Sweet potatoes contain half the sugar and four times the mineral content of regular white potatoes, so for anyone wishing to upgrade their diet, but not ready to leave potatoes off the menu, this is a good place to begin. Please see the recipe section for some tasty and satisfying meals that are based on root vegetables, including sweet potatoes.

Fruit

Moving on to fruit, which seems a natural progression from vegetables, we generally observe that fruit crosses the boundary between alkaline and acidic residue. It is worth mentioning here that there is often confusion about lemons. Lemons, like all citrus fruit, contain citric acid, so are often labelled as acid-forming as a result. However, it isn't as simple as that. Lemons, once digested, leave an alkaline mineral residue despite their citric acid content, so are usually considered to be an alkaline fruit.

Ripe tropical fruits are an excellent food. Our main challenge in the Western world, however, is that it is almost impossible to obtain ripe tropical fruit – you really would have to consider moving to the tropics if you wanted to alkalise your body in this way. Overconsumption of unripe fruit is one of the fastest ways in which to aggravate bone loss. Allow me to explain. Although fruit is considered by many to be a true health food, most if not all the fruit that reaches our northern shores is picked prior to peak ripeness. This is problematic because the greatest mineralisation occurs just before full ripeness, and the fruit cannot be picked at this stage since it would spoil during shipment. Another complication of fruit is that it is very often hybridised, which almost by definition now means that it is high in sugar and low in minerals, two more aggravating factors for osteoporosis. Dr Brian Clement, director of the Hippocrates Health Institute in Florida, notes that the population group with the second highest incidence of osteoporosis is the high fruit eaters who do not exercise. The highest incidence is found in the high meat eaters who do not exercise. For reversing osteoporosis, if you do not happen to live in the tropics, I therefore recommend that you keep your fruit consumption to a minimum and focus on the lower glycaemic fruits, so as not to aggravate bone loss via excess acidic load.

Sprouted grains

There is a lot of controversy surrounding grains, and not just in the health food community. Some authors are vehement in their condemnation of grains of all types, whilst others see them as a very balancing food, especially the small alkalising or neutral sprouted grains such as quinoa, amaranth and teff. I feel that we should not be 'tarring all grains with the same brush'. Modern-day wheat is a poor grain choice and it is known to be highly hybridised, containing vast amounts of gluten which sticks to our intestinal wall and is considered to be responsible for many health issues, including widespread allergies. People affected by coeliac disease (an aggressive manifestation of gluten intolerance) are known to have a higher incidence of osteoporosis than the general population, and are prone to multiple nutritional deficiencies. When placed on gluten-free diets, these people's bone density improves. Another good reason to go gluten-free is that standard hybridised wheat is high in phytates, compounds that can bind minerals such as calcium and prevent them from being absorbed. Many authors teach us that cooked hybridised grains are also highly addictive and cause an undesirable alteration in brain chemistry.

It's not all bad news. By sprouting the small alkaline or neutral residue grains we have a gluten-free food that not only does not aggravate osteoporosis, but also contains many other elements that are beneficial for health; for example vitamin content, which I discuss in more detail in chapter 9. In the recipe section you'll find plenty of ideas for some great meals that incorporate the small, healthy grains. Cut out the wheat, but enjoy quinoa, amaranth and buckwheat (which is not strictly a grain, but a member of the rhubarb family).

Now let's move on to the things that will tip the body more towards acidity, and therefore aggravate demineralisation of the bones. These are the 'bad guys'.

The 'bad guys'

Nuts and seeds

Nuts and seeds are the most dense of the foods that are used in a plant-based diet. They are high-protein, high-fat foods and my recommendation is that they should be used sparingly, and always soaked or sprouted prior to consumption. Nuts and seeds leave an acidic residue, which is fine if they are balanced with a diet that is very high in the alkalising green leaves. As long as the diet is mostly made up of greens, a small quantity of soaked seeds and nuts can be used daily as a good vegan protein source and as a beneficial source of essential fatty acids for hormone balance, which is also discussed later in chapter 11. In the recipe section you will find some nut- and seed-based dishes that will satisfy even the most discerning palate.

Meat

Meat leaves a highly acidic residue since it is a high-protein substance that has a predominance of phosphorus, nitrogen, sulphur, carbon and hydrogen. The microcrystalline matrix of bone contains phosphorus, but it has to be in balance with calcium in a ratio of two to one in favour of calcium. The acidity of meat cannot be balanced out by eating raw green leaves – we would not be able to physically consume a sufficient quantity of leaves if meat were to be eaten daily. In studies performed on unfortunate people who decided to follow the Atkins diet, it was found that after only six months on this disastrous diet, their urinary calcium excretion increased by 50 per cent. Increased urinary calcium excretion associated with animal protein consumption has been known for over 80 years. We will talk more about this when we come onto the protein section in chapter 5, but for now suffice it to say that meat is acidic and must be avoided by anyone who is serious about building bone strength.

Sugar and all processed carbohydrates

I have devoted another complete chapter to this topic, so likewise will discuss the sugar and carbohydrate story in more detail in chapter 6. For now, remember that all processed food of this type, particularly cakes, biscuits, pastries, bread and anything containing processed white refined flour, are acidic and will aggravate osteoporosis and facilitate bone loss.

Alcohol

Alcohol always leaves an acidic residue in the body and aggravates many conditions. It has no place in the health seeker's diet. Alcohol has been proven over time to be a potent destroyer of bone structure. Alcoholics have a four-times greater incidence of osteoporosis than the normal population. In addition to rotting the bones, it causes considerable damage to liver and brain cells, as I discuss in my previous book *The Whole Body Solution*. For reversing osteoporosis, alcohol must be avoided; you'll find more information about this issue in chapter 10.

Fizzy/carbonated drinks

Fizzy drinks, sodas, cola; whatever you like to call them, they will have a massive impact on your acid/alkali balance. Would you really, should you be so invited, drink a glass of phosphoric acid? Of course you wouldn't (unless someone dared you to and you wanted to prove something). So why drink a can of cola? Read the list of ingredients, and you will see that in addition to water, sugar and caramel, it's there for all to see – phosphoric acid. It is accepted as a controversial food additive, called E338, and it is evidently cheaper to add to food than is citric acid. I really am at a loss to understand why anyone would want to add phosphoric acid to anything, apart from maybe a car battery. It is used in industrial applications as a rust remover. Do our digestive systems contain rust? Not that I am aware of.

Not only does phosphoric acid understandably make our tissues more acidic, and therefore increase the need for alkaline minerals to counteract this undesirable situation, it also has the interesting property of binding with calcium and magnesium in the digestive tract, so that any beneficial sources of calcium and magnesium consumed within three hours of the can of drink would be completely negated. Studies have shown that those who consume large quantities of acidic fizzy drinks have lower bone density than the general population. A counter-suggestion which has been put forward, rather weakly in relation to phosphoric acid, is that phosphorus intake is necessary for strong bones because phosphorus is present in bones. As mentioned above this is true, but we cannot utilise phosphoric acid, and it has no benefit for bone strength. This counter argument should be dismissed as nonsense – it was funded by a cola manufacturer.

It takes 32 cans of water to dilute out the chemical nastiness of one can of cola. Do you see schoolchildren walking to school with 32 cans of water in a large rucksack as they go along with that red can in their hand? Of course not. Most canned carbonated drinks contain approximately 12 teaspoons of sugar. We will be talking about refined white sugar in more detail later, but the phosphoric acid, sugar and caffeine (caffeine causes calcium loss from bones) present should alert one to the possibility that this is not appropriate stuff to be drinking.

Leave a tooth overnight in a glass containing cola and all traces of that tooth will be gone by morning. Tooth enamel is the hardest substance in the human body. It is not designed to disappear overnight! Police in the USA on road duty carry large bottles of cola with them. Sensibly they do not drink it, but use it to rapidly rid the roads of blood after car crashes. I also hear that it is particularly useful for cleaning toilets.

Let us not, dear reader, add to the already bulging coffers of companies that profit from a product that has only harmful effects on our health. Do not be fooled into thinking that the 'diet' version of any of these drinks is less damaging. They still contain phosphoric acid. They still contain caffeine. They do not contain sugar, but they almost universally will contain aspartame, one of the most controversial and horrifically damaging additives ever to appear in the food supply. For more information on the dreadful bodily effects of aspartame, and its chemical relative acesulfame-K, please refer to my CD 'Feeding the Brain', available at www.therawfoodscientist.com, or do your own internet search.

Finally, if you needed any other reasons never to buy a canned drink again, those who consume liquids out of cans are increasing their exposure to toxic aluminium by up to six times. In addition to being linked to Alzheimer's disease, aluminium reduces the formation of the bone matrix and, if that weren't enough, increases the rate of bone resorption, both of which in turn increase our overall fracture risk.[5]

Caffeine

Present of course in the aforementioned carbonated drinks but also in something that most people seem to need in the mornings to get them going – coffee. Coffee is a universally accepted substance and some researchers even (maybe in desperation) claim that it has health benefits, citing that it contains antioxidants. It is a drug. It causes increased tissue acidity. It causes adrenal stress (as if we didn't have enough of that in our lives already), and it causes demineralisation of bones not only by increasing the urinary excretion of calcium, but also by blocking its absorption. Numerous research papers have indicated a positive correlation between increased caffeine intake and the increased likelihood of hip fracture. There is really no need for any more scientific studies to be performed on coffee, we already know from previous research that it's damaging. Coffee and all caffeinated drinks reduce bone strength and must be avoided to enable us to adequately restructure the skeleton.

It can be hard cutting out coffee; after all, it is an addictive substance. Do it gradually to avoid the withdrawal headaches that often present themselves, and get to bed earlier so that you do not feel the need for artificial stimulants to get you going. Or alternatively, just bite the bullet and go cold turkey. It doesn't really matter how you eliminate the stuff, just make sure that you do it.

I was recently amused to read in a so-called 'health' article that because doctors are aware that coffee aggravates bone loss, their recommendation is to limit consumption to no more than three cups per day, and to make sure that you add some milk to your coffee to offset the calcium loss that caffeine causes. In other words, your daily 'latte' is good for you! To me, this advice is ridiculous. We know, for example, that smoking causes death and also bone destruction (see below), but are doctors recommending that you only smoke half a pack per day rather than a full pack? Of course not. I am not going to tell you what you want to hear, I'm telling you what you need to hear. Coffee is responsible for bone loss; you should therefore stop drinking it. Cutting down is a poor substitute for cutting out. And from what you have learned in chapter 3, you will be aware that adding milk to coffee will do your bones no favours whatsoever.

Before you ask, decaffeinated products are not the answer either. They can contain up to 97 per cent of the caffeine present in the original product (yes, amazingly, it can be called decaffeinated even if only 3 per cent of the caffeine has been removed), and the decaffeination process itself utilises turpentine and embalming fluid (a known carcinogen), with some residues invariably being present in the 'decaffeinated' end product.

Please remember that the many of the so-called 'healthy treat' foods, such as raw chocolate, also contain caffeine. Some authors describe raw chocolate as a health food due to its high ORAC (oxygen radical absorption capacity) value, meaning that it contains good levels of antioxidants. Indeed it does, but the fact that it also contains caffeine, and is often used in combination with sugar and fat to make desserts, render it a potentially bone demineralising food, despite the fact that it contains good levels of magnesium, which you can read about in chapter 8.

Smoking

If ever there were a reason not to smoke, it is for the sake of bone health. In addition to all of the other extremely well-documented dangers of this noxious and carcinogenic habit, smoking causes an acidic state in the body. However, smoking appears to tip us temporarily towards a more alkaline state, because it delivers alkaloids which 'fool' the body into thinking it is becoming more alkaline. The effect however is very short lived, lasting an hour at the most, and then the body ends up being more acidic than it was before. As a result, cravings are then manifested for the next 'alkaline fix', and the negative spiral starts all over again.

Additionally, smoking also delivers high levels of the toxic heavy metal cadmium into the body. Cadmium is well known to weaken the bones.[6]

Depending on the research you read, smokers have an approximately three times greater incidence of osteoporosis than non-smokers. Whether your concern is heart disease, cancer, osteoporosis or more rapid ageing, the facts are clear that smoking promotes them all. Eliminate this dangerous habit from your life if you have not already done so, and feel the difference.

Do other methods of alkalising the body work?

Many people are now enjoying the 'health benefits' of other methods that are 'proven' to alkalise the body, so that you don't have to go to the effort of changing your diet. In other words, keep doing everything that is bad for you, and just take 'product A' or 'product B' instead. Ah, if only it were that simple; and how sad it is that everyone wants a quick fix. Anything worthwhile is worth working hard for. If we want good health, and strong bones, we have to put in some effort.

'Alkaline water'

I have been offered, and enjoyed, 'pH 9' water in numerous

health-conscious restaurants and whilst it tasted fine, I have to say I was always sceptical, having received a good grounding in basic chemistry. I became more sceptical still when someone tried to tell me that my life would not be complete, and my health would not be optimal, unless I invested in a water ioniser for £4000 which produced alkaline water. Allow me to elaborate.

The pH of water is determined by three factors: temperature, dissolved gases and mineral content. Water is what is known as a 'weakly buffered' solution, meaning that it cannot easily resist changes to its pH, neither can it change the pH of a strongly buffered solution (such as, for example, hydrochloric acid) to a great degree. Therefore, as soon as alkaline water enters the stomach, which contains hydrochloric acid, a 'true' acid, it immediately becomes neutralised. Even if we did want to change the acidity of our stomach, alkaline water won't do it. As it turns out, we don't want to dilute our pH in the stomach, because we need a good level of stomach acidity to help us to assimilate many of the minerals that we need for good bone health. Therefore, drinking alkaline water will not make a difference to the pH of your blood or your cells, although, on the face of it, it does seem to be a nice idea.

I'd invest the £4000 elsewhere, especially since studies involving rats have indicated that long-term use of alkaline water causes pathological changes in the muscles of the heart, and potentially dangerous elevations in blood potassium levels.[7]

'Alkaline' oral sprays

'The hottest breakthrough nutritional sprays the industry has ever seen' reads the bold claim on one particular website. Their 'miraculous' alkalising oral spray is, apparently, 'particularly beneficial for the thousands of people who are trying to make their bodies alkaline and find it difficult adjusting to a restricted diet or changing their lifestyle.' Again, those seeking a 'quick fix' are unlikely to find one. For your US$25 or so for one small bottle, this product will not actually give you any particular health benefits, despite the company's overinflated claims, since the ingredients are little more than chalk and chlorophyll. There's nothing wrong with chlorophyll, and there is plenty of it in wheatgrass juice – a far better source than this particular product or any other that makes similar claims. 'pH drops' are likewise of dubious value despite aggressive promotion in some health fields.

There is no 'quick fix' for alkalising your body to protect your bones. Maintaining an ideal acid / alkali balance in the body comes from following the advice given throughout this book, and loving your bones enough to want to do the best for them in the long term. If that means a total lifestyle and diet change, then so be it. However, if I do ever find a quick fix that has been scientifically proven to work, you can be sure I'll be writing about it.

Chapter 4 summary

- Our blood has to stay at a slightly alkaline pH to maintain life.
- Food leaves either an acidic or alkaline residue in the body. The most alkaline-forming foods are those which are best for bone health and should be eaten in abundance; these include green vegetable juices and green salad leaves.
- Coffee, canned fizzy drinks and alcohol are some of the worst offenders for aggravating bone loss.
- Smoking leads to increased tissue acidity and closely correlates with increased fracture risk.
- The only way in which we can alkalise the body is via excellent food choices. Other methods are useless at best and potentially harmful at worst.

Chapter 5

Protein damage and unhealthy doctors

Considerable interest always seems to be generated over the premature death of those famous for writing books on health, diet and weight loss. One would anticipate that, particularly in relation to authors of weight-loss books, they must themselves be lean and healthy. This is often far from the case. The post mortem results for Dr Atkins, who gave his name to the infamous diet that he created, were kept secret for a number of years because they may have exposed the diet for what it was – a disaster for health and wellbeing. We are intelligent people; let us therefore consider the following. If something is good for us, we should be able to do it for our whole lives and obtain only benefits from doing it. If something is harmful, and we are not recommended to be able to do it for the rest of our lives but only in the short term, how can it possibly be perceived to have any benefits? But so it was with the Atkins diet – a 'quick fix' for weight loss that was not recommended for long-term use. When the eagerly awaited post mortem results became publicly available, it was noted that Dr Atkins was bordering on obese and had confirmed heart disease. So his recommended diet didn't even work for him.

As I state in my CD 'The Real Truth about Food', available through my website www.therawfoodscientist.com, I like to judge by results. If anyone who is fat is telling you how you should lose weight, I would be inclined to look elsewhere for advice. Would you, for example, take 'how to stop smoking' classes from a smoker? Of course not. I recommend that you seek out the people who are getting the results you are looking for, and find out what they are doing.

Good and bad proteins for bones

So that's the unhealthy doctors part covered, but you might be wondering what all this has to do with protein and, in turn, bone health. Quite simply, although protein is a necessary part of our diet, it can cause collateral damage when eaten to excess. It has been estimated that in the USA, there are 300,000,000 people suffering from the adverse effects of excess protein consumption (cancer, heart disease, diabetes, arthritis and osteoporosis), and only a handful of people who might have true protein deficiency. True protein deficiency, medically referred to as kwashiorkor, is incredibly rare, and is generally confined to famine-ridden parts of Africa.

Not all proteins are created equal, however. Animal-derived proteins are considerably more acidic in nature than plant proteins,[1] increasing the acidic load in the body. A further large-scale study has indicated a strong correlation between animal protein consumption and bone fracture rate in women in various countries.[2] Animal protein also contributes to an increase in individual risk of cancer and heart disease, whereas plant protein consumption does not. For fascinating research into the detrimental effects of animal protein consumption, I recommend reading *The China Study* by T. Colin Campbell.

In addition to being acidic, and therefore throwing our pH out of whack, animal proteins have been demonstrated to inhibit the production of a particularly active form of vitamin D.[3] Vitamin D, together with its vitally important role in bone health, is discussed in considerably more detail in chapter 9. For now, we may know it as the vitamin that gives us strong bones, since a deficiency of it in childhood leads to rickets, common in 19th-century England in children that were forced to work long hours in factories, and as a result never saw the light of day.

When looking at protein consumption in general, it is interesting to look at the ratio between animal protein and plant protein in the diet. Studies across several countries have indicated that the further the balance is tipped in favour of plant protein, and the less animal protein is consumed, the lower the incidence of hip fracture.[4] Hip fracture is probably the best indicator of bone strength, since, as previously mentioned, high BMD (bone mineral density) does not always correlate precisely with a reduced incidence of hip fracture.

The further we move towards all of our dietary protein coming from plants, the less likely hip fractures become. In Nigeria, the animal to plant protein ratio is 10 per cent that of the average European country, and their incidence of hip fracture is just 1 per cent of ours. Maybe this helps to explain why dairy products contribute to osteoporosis, since they are a high-protein, animal-derived food. Some studies have shown that meat eaters have a higher incidence of osteoporosis later in life than that found in vegetarians, whilst others have shown no significant difference. Could it be that the vegetarian participants in the negative studies had a high dairy intake? I will leave you to draw your own conclusions; I have already drawn mine.

In the past there have been concerns raised that a plant-based diet does not contain adequate protein to sustain humans, and in my previous book, *The Whole Body Solution*, I went into further detail about this particular concern. The theory, popularised in the 1970s, that we need to 'combine' proteins for adequate amino acid intake has been disproven, and people eating a wide variety of plant foods, particularly if they are regularly consuming sprouted greens, have no need to worry about their protein intake.

For readers who are used to basing their diet on meals which include meat, it can be difficult to know where to begin, and just leaving out meat from your diet can potentially leave you confused as to what you should eat instead. I am recommending a plant-based diet, but what, in a practical sense, does this involve? Substitution and upgrading are the key. Mushrooms, for example, give a 'meaty' texture to meals. The small grains, as described in chapter 4, contain reasonable amounts of protein. Pulses, such as lentils and chick peas, are also good sources of vegetable protein. Nuts and sunflower seeds are the most dense plant proteins and will leave you satisfied. I have divided the recipe section into dishes based on all these ingredients, so that you will have the option for plenty of variety in your plant-based meal choices.

Chapter 5 summary

- Protein from animal sources is detrimental to bone health.
- Meat consumption creates an unfavourable acidic load in the body.
- Animal protein consumption interferes with vitamin D metabolism, adversely affecting bone strength.

Chapter 6

Sugar – the 4th deadly sin

Sugar consumption in the Western world has reached an all-time high while the incidence of osteoporosis in the Western world seems also to be increasing exponentially. Could there be a link in this alarming situation? The sugar industry will no doubt disagree, and say that it is pure coincidence; indeed, there are other interesting 'trends' that we can find which are completely unrelated to each other, such as the odd one that I heard about recently, in which the divorce rate was found to be inversely proportional to the purchase of margarine. It really is amazing what some people study, isn't it? Sugar consumption, however, can have a significant impact on bone integrity. Here is my take on the sugar story.

Adrenaline and stress hormones

Sugar, and high-sugar foods such as cakes, biscuits and all those other snacks that I would place in the 'non-food' category, increase acidity as I have already mentioned, and have been shown to increase urinary calcium excretion. High-sugar diets also increase adrenaline production fourfold. If we are continuously being affected by adrenaline, which puts the body into a high-stress, 'fear, fight, flight' mode, we increase our acidity further and run alkaline minerals out of the body, as well as revving up the metabolism to allow us to escape from imminent danger. However, there is no imminent danger, apart from that of the sugar consumption itself.

Consumption of refined sugar increases the production of cortisol, another stress hormone, which in turn has detrimental effects on bone strength. This effect is considered to be as a result of cortisol's inhibition of DHEA (dehydroepiandrosterone), a hormone which promotes bone building. I will discuss this in more detail later on, in the hormone section in chapter 11. This undesirable effect of cortisol is well known by the medical profession, and is one of the reasons why doctors do not tend to prescribe corticosteroids indiscriminately, since they are well documented to be a contributory factor in osteoporosis.

Sugar also interferes with the transport of, and functions of, vitamin C. As we will see in chapters 8 and 9, when I discuss the vitamins and minerals which are necessary for bone health, vitamin C plays an important part in the formation of strong healthy bone tissue.

Diabetic dangers

It is now being increasingly recognised that the bones of diabetics are weaker than those of non-diabetics. Small-scale studies conducted by the Mayo Clinic have indicated that diabetics have a 12 per cent reduction of bone strength in comparison with non-diabetics, and are at greater risk of fractures as a result. Diabetic complications are a result of elevated blood glucose, and those consuming a high-sugar diet can push themselves quite easily into a state of temporary diabetes as a result of their food choices. The exact mechanism of damage to bone caused by high-sugar intake, or the diabetic state, is not fully known, but researchers at the Mayo Clinic have postulated that it is a result of a type of molecule known as an AGE. AGE is an acronym for advanced glycation end-product. Don't worry too much about the name.

AGEs occur when sugar combines with a protein molecule, and they really do AGE you! In the case of bone, sugar combines with the collagen matrix of the bone, which affects how the bone cells function, with the overall effect being that of bone weakening.

Excess fruit and ready meals

Those following a so-called 'healthy diet' are not automatically immune from the dangers of sugar. Adherents of a wholefood, unprocessed dietary regime are no doubt doing themselves a huge favour, but that does not automatically mean that the diet is low in sugar. Many hybridised (and that includes seedless) fruits are high in sugar and low in minerals, so if your 'healthy' diet includes a lot of hybridised sweet fruit and not enough greens and sprouted food, you are potentially in as much danger from osteoporosis as the average 'meat and two vegetables' eater.

The sugar content of food may not be immediately obvious. Sugar is used as a flavour enhancer, and in many processed 'ready meals' the sugar content can be alarmingly high, as it is in condiments such as shop-bought salad dressings. Even for those following a diet low in processed foods, many 'healthy' dessert recipes can also contain alarming quantities of added sugar in the form of date paste, agave syrup (now known to be particularly unhealthy for other reasons, notably its fructose content), maple syrup and other such ingredients. Just because it is 'unprocessed' doesn't mean it's healthy. Ensure you are one of the whole-food eaters that doesn't rely on, for example, raw cakes, 'treat foods' and the like to fill you up with calories. The best wholefood diet for strong bones is always going to be that based on greens, greens and more greens.

Other dangers associated with sugar consumption

A diet high in refined sugar really is a recipe for disaster, not only from the point of view of bone health. Whilst researching for a presentation I gave in 2010, which later became one of my CD and MP3 recordings entitled '*The Dangers of Excess Sugar Consumption*', I uncovered the following facts:

Addictions

Sugar is an addictive substance and can be as difficult to eliminate as hard drugs. It affects the brain chemicals beta endorphin and serotonin. Serotonin is one of our 'happy hormones', and initially sugar makes us feel happy, but soon after we get the reverse, and therefore need another 'fix' to get us going again. It has been stated that high sugar intake can lead to an increased incidence of alcoholism, and it is well known that all alcoholics have an underlying blood sugar regulation problem.[1] The way in which fructose (fruit sugar) affects the liver is similar to the way alcohol affects it. Some even state that fructose is alcohol without the buzz, since its metabolic pathway is different from that of sucrose (table sugar). Alcohol in relation to bone health is discussed further in chapter 10.

Ageing

Now, let's get onto vanity. Sugar causes accelerated ageing, as a result of excessive cross-linking of proteins, which lead to increased wrinkling of the skin and, as a result of mineral depletion, grey hair. Now of course you can go down the face lift, hair dye and botox route. But might it not be preferable to eat better? It is certainly cheaper and much healthier. As mentioned above, an area of research which is being given much attention recently is the tendency of some types of food to cause AGEs. Processed carbohydrates such as baked goods and processed sugars such as high fructose corn syrup are high in AGEs and contribute to chronic inflammation, free radical damage and a propensity towards diabetes and kidney damage. AGEs formed when sugar binds to animal protein and fat are known to be particularly dangerous.

Arthritis

In addition to undermining bone health, sugar adversely affects the joints, aggravating arthritis. This is generally considered to be due to increased acidity, but can also be attributable to increased oxidative damage to the joints, since sugar increases free radical damage to many bodily tissues.[2] Sugar also causes our tendons to become brittle. That is certainly not a desirable situation for anyone, but is especially problematic if you participate in competitive sports.

Cancer

Sugar feeds cancer cells. Every time we consume sugar, it causes an insulin spike, whereby insulin is secreted from the pancreas to drive sugar into the cells to keep the blood glucose levels constant. The cells with the most insulin receptors, i.e. cancer cells, which require approximately 20 times more glucose than normal cells, grab the glucose and feed first. Prolonged high insulin levels, according to the research biochemist Dr Mitra Ray,[3] have been shown to correlate strongly with cancer. Harvard Medical School also concluded that girls who eat a lot of sugar early in life have a much greater risk of breast cancer later in life.

Dementia

Sugar is also suggested to play a part in the onset of vascular dementia, via its effect on the body of increasing uric acid.[4] This is mostly attributed to the effects of fructose, and it is stated that, for optimal health, we should eat no more than 25 g of fructose per day. Increased levels of uric acid also increase the risks of obesity, heart disease, hypertension, stroke and kidney disease. Fructose is not alone in causing dangerously high levels of uric acid, since consumption of meat also plays a part. The human body can only process approximately 8 g of uric acid per day, whereas an average serving of meat contains 16 g. If we combine a high-sugar (fructose) diet with meat eating, we really are inviting some serious future trouble.

Dental disease

You don't need me to remind you about this one; I'm sure your dentist has been telling you that sweets and sugar are bad for your teeth for as long as you can remember. However, despite all the evidence, there are still some authorities who would have you believe that the best way to avoid dental caries is to brush your teeth with toothpaste that contains fluoride, and consume cheese. Recent studies however seem to indicate that fluoride in toothpaste has no beneficial effect on dental health, and the recommendation about fluoride and cheese quoted above comes from Sugar Nutrition UK, whose mission statement is 'Improving knowledge and understanding about the contributions of sugar and other carbohydrates to a healthy balanced diet'. One of their chief scientists is part of the scientific and communications committee of the World Sugar Research Organisation, which in turn is funded by the sugar industry. I'll leave you to work out the implications of that association for yourself; it shouldn't take you long.

DNA damage

As mentioned above, sugar increases free radical production in the body, and this can in turn lead to DNA damage, notably by exerting an effect on the protein structure of DNA.[5] Free radicals have such widespread detrimental effects on the body that we need to minimise them in every way that we can; after all, they are now considered to be one of the primary causes of degenerative disease and ageing. Fortunately, a plant-based diet which is high in natural antioxidants, as discussed in later chapters, tips the balance very much in our favour.

Heart disease

Heart disease is the most common killer in the UK, but it is being rapidly chased by cancer. These two degenerative diseases are closely linked to consumption of high levels of processed carbohydrates,[6] and animal protein; yet another reason why I advocate a plant-based diet. Sugar not only contributes to atherosclerosis, which is hardening of the arteries, but also makes our platelets more sticky, which in turn increases the likelihood of a stroke.

After a 15-year study, Harvard Medical School concluded that people who obtain 25 per cent of their calories from sugar are more than twice as likely to die from cardiovascular disease, regardless of their body mass index. However, the opinion of the World Sugar Research Organisation is somewhat different. Funded by those with a vested interest, and echoed by Sugar Nutrition UK, their statement on the issue, revised in 2013, is as follows:

> *In agreement with many reviews undertaken by international bodies, we do not consider that there is convincing evidence of any relationship between sugar intake and direct or indirect risk of cardiovascular disease.*

Is it any wonder that the public remains confused as to what we should base the diet upon?

Hormonal disruption

Women seem to suffer more than men with hormonal imbalances, and by the time we reach about the age of 35, our hormonal balance can be significantly affected. Women who eat a high-sugar diet suffer more with PMS,[7] and additionally have a problem with oestrogen dominance, which I highlight in chapter 11. For more information on oestrogen dominance, its negative effects on health and what to do about it, please read my previous book *The Whole Body Solution*.

Obesity

Obesity is at an all-time high, as is our sugar consumption. Obesity is one of the most preventable diseases there is, and one of the best ways to defend against it is to eliminate refined sugar, particularly fructose, which is hiding in many processed foods. Fructose disrupts the stimulation of a hormone called leptin, which is the satiety hormone – in other words, leptin is your friend because it makes you feel full. By consuming a lot of sugar, and in particular fructose, the trigger to stopping eating is switched off, so that people end up inadvertently consuming more. It is not as simple as the original 'calories in, calories out' model; obesity is a complex disease, with inactivity being a major component of the problem. However, sugar consumption is an important part of the overall picture, despite what Sugar Nutrition UK, and the sugar industry in general, would like you to believe.

Chapter 6 summary

- Sugar is detrimental to bone health as a result of increasing both acidic load and adrenal stress.
- Those eating a lot of processed carbohydrates, including but not limited to white flour, pasta, pastries, cakes, candies and sweets, are putting themselves at greater risk of poor bone health.
- Eating too much sweet fruit can also be detrimental to bone health.

- Hidden sugars are present in many processed foods, such as convenience meals, and should be avoided.
- High sugar consumption is linked to many other disease processes, including, but not limited to, more rapid ageing, cancer, dental disease, dementia, hormonal disruption and obesity.

Chapter 7

Calcium – less important than you may think

It's all we ever hear about in relation to bones, isn't it? And it's the question I am always asked when people hear that I have been dairy-free for over 35 years: 'Where do you get your calcium?' So it might surprise you to know that I really don't place great importance on calcium. Indeed, our intake of calcium is of secondary importance. What is much more important is the rate at which we lose it; that is, our overall calcium balance.

Lessons from South Africa

Have you heard of the Bantu Africans? You may not have done, but they are remarkable in relation to their bone strength and calcium intake. What are we being told here in the UK about our recommended calcium intake? Have you heard that we should be having between 1000 mg and 1200 mg of calcium every day, and if we don't reach that intake level we need to take inorganic calcium pills, generally made of chalk and therefore not bioavailable in the slightest? In the USA, the recommended daily allowance for calcium is set even higher, at 1500 mg per day. Let's consider the South African Bantu women. They are tall, have wonderful jaw structure and straight white teeth, and they often have up to 10 children, all of whom are breastfed. They have a practically zero incidence of osteoporosis, even in advanced age. It might surprise you to hear, therefore, that their daily intake of calcium is a mere 300 mg, and some researchers have therefore questioned whether the present insistence on high calcium intake is justified.[1]

How do the Bantu do it? They are simply not exposed to the calcium loss that we are. One of the reasons that our RDA is set so high is because we are literally passing out our bones with our urine, as a result of our meat- and dairy-based, highly acidic diet and poor lifestyle choices.

Other studies have suggested that calcium intake in adult middle-aged female subjects seems to make little to no difference as to whether those women are likely to sustain a fracture. Indeed, researchers in Sweden concluded that dietary calcium or vitamin D intakes estimated at middle and older age do not seem to be of major importance in the primary prevention of osteoporotic fractures in women.[2] I cover vitamin D later on, in chapter 9, and state that the best source of this nutrient is via sun exposure, rather than via diet, so perhaps this research conclusion is unsurprising.

High-calcium eggshells from low-calcium hens

Years ago, scientists were initially baffled when they discovered that egg-laying hens on a low calcium diet continued to produce egg shells with a higher calcium content than the diet contained. How was this possible? Where was that extra calcium coming from? Welcome to the fascinating world of C. Louis Kervran (1901-1983), who wrote about the concept of biological transmutations. This modern-day alchemy describes the body's potential ability to transform one element into another, and, according to Kervran, explains why 'calcium-deficient' hens can continue to lay eggs with strong, calcium-rich shells, and additionally why Sahara oilfield workers were found to be able to excrete 320 mg more calcium than they were consuming without bone decalcification[3]. Indeed, some authors are indicating that we should be treating hip fractures with a low-calcium diet, a recommendation which seems to fly completely in the face of conventional thinking.

Whether or not biological transmutations are possible inside the human body is currently debatable, and no other scientists seem to have followed up on Kervran's work. Such transmutations are possible in physical experiments during which high temperatures are used, but whether it is possible at the temperature of the human body is unknown, and a little outside the scope of this particular book. It does, however, pose interesting questions about whether we have overstated the importance of calcium intake in relation to bone health. For post-menopausal women, the protein:calcium ratio (i.e. how much protein is consumed in relation to how much calcium) appears to be a better predictor of fracture risk than calcium intake alone.[4]

Misleading X-rays?

The reason that so much emphasis is placed on calcium is that it is the mineral which makes up most of our bone structure, and therefore is considered to be vital for bone mineral density (BMD) as measured via bone scans. Calcium is a hard tissue that shows up well on X-ray and DEXA scanning, so if there is a greater deposition of calcium in the bones, they show up as being denser on the scan, so the conclusion is drawn that the bone must therefore be stronger. However, we need to bear in mind that X-rays and DEXA scans don't actually give much indication of the tensile strength of the bone – that is, how it responds when force is applied to it. As I have mentioned previously, in chapter 2, BMD is not an altogether accurate determinant of fracture risk. Indeed, there are certain parts of the world in which overall bone mass and BMD are lower than in developed nations, but the fracture rate is also lower. As mentioned previously, a better predictor of osteoporosis is the dietary ratio of plant protein to animal protein, and BMD is not significantly associated with this ratio.[5]

The case against calcium

It has now been shown that taking large doses of calcium as a single mineral supplement can actually cause considerable harm, and may make no real impact on the rate of bone loss. Many of the supplements produced by the pharmaceutical industry and recommended to doctors to prescribe to their patients have no clinical studies to support their use. This was demonstrated to me recently during a conversation with someone I met who was a drugs rep (now, I believe, called a 'territory manager') for a pharmaceutical company. I asked her what her role was in the company, and she replied: 'I sell calcium supplements to doctors.'

This immediately got my attention, and I wanted to know more. I asked where the clinical trials, involving the particular supplement which her company produced, were published. She looked surprised. 'Clinical trials? For what?' Well, clinical trials showing evidence of reduced fracture risk when taking the supplement she was promoting, I continued. Her response was shocking, although perhaps I should have been prepared for the answer. 'Oh, there aren't any trials for our supplement. But we all know that bones are made of calcium, so if you take calcium supplements you won't get osteoporosis.'

This, in my opinion, is almost as daft as saying that bones are white and milk is white, so milk must therefore be good for bones. Is this really the extent of the 'anti-osteoporosis' education that doctors are receiving? How about asking for some decent science to back up the recommendations? Large doses of calcium, especially in a non-bioavailable form (i.e. an individual isolated supplement, not made from wholefood but made, usually, from chalk) can interfere with the absorption and utilisation of other minerals; for example iron, zinc, and more importantly in relation to bone strength, magnesium. As we will see in the next chapter, magnesium could be considered to be more important than calcium when it comes to building healthy bone structure.

Chapter 7

Food, not pills, with one exception

In summary, yes we do need calcium, but our best source of this mineral is always going to be from food, rather than via inorganic supplementation. Kale is an excellent source (raw or juiced), and many other greens, including watercress, lamb's lettuce, red clover sprouts and Chinese cabbage (bok choi) contain good quantities. I like to use raw tahini in sauces and smoothies, since it contains a good level of bioavailable calcium, as well as being a great source of plant protein. Hemp seeds are another good source of calcium, in addition to being a very health-giving food. Green juices, made from green leaves and low-glycaemic vegetables such as cucumber and celery, will contain all the daily calcium that you might need. You'll find a fantastic green juice recipe in my book *The Whole Body Solution*, and I have also included it at the end of this book in Appendix 1, because, in my opinion, it is so important to overall health.

In addition to its role in bone health, calcium is also necessary for other biological processes. It is vital for the correct functioning of nerves and muscles, including the regulation of the heartbeat. It also plays a role in the blood-clotting cascade (the chain of events from injury to blood clot formation) and the release of hormones and other chemicals. We should access all the calcium we need for bone health via a healthy plant-based diet, and I certainly do not recommend supplementing with inorganic calcium tablets (calcium carbonate or calcium citrate).

'Chalk-based' inorganic calcium supplements have now definitely been superseded by a full-spectrum, whole plant-based mineral supplement called AlgaeCal, which has been shown in clinical trials to have far more impressive results in the stimulation of osteoblast activity and proliferation.[6] It was demonstrated in this study that AlgaeCal increased the number of human bone building cells by 400 per cent more than calcium carbonate. The study findings provided evidence that AlgaeCal plant calcium is superior to the two most popular forms of calcium in all test parameters – the first time in the history of calcium research that a significant difference was shown between the many commercially available calcium ingredients' effect on bone cells. Safety studies have also indicated no detrimental or adverse effects from this type of wholefood supplementation.[7]

I have no affiliations with the company that produces AlgaeCal, but for bone health, I do recommend a particular supplement into which AlgaeCal is incorporated. This is a product called 'Source of Life Garden Bone Support', made by Nature's Plus. It is the only 'calcium' supplement that I will ever recommend for bone health, and that is fundamentally because it isn't actually a calcium supplement; it is a full mineral wholefood product which also incorporates magnesium, vitamin D, vitamin K2 and other vital nutrients for bone health that you'll read about in following chapters.

Dangers of non-wholefood calcium supplementation

Heart attack risks

A Swedish cohort study, which followed participants for three years, indicated a 24 per cent increase in all-cause mortality in those taking calcium supplements. The risk of heart attacks increased, but that of stroke did not. These findings correlated to population groups studied elsewhere, according to the results of a German study involving almost 24,000 people, followed for over a decade. This study, despite being described as 'flawed' by a doctor representing the Health Supplements Information Service (which is funded by supplement manufacturers, so will not be unbiased), found that there was an 86 per cent increase in the risk of heart attacks in the supplemented group compared with those who did not take the inorganic calcium.

This study has sparked a vigorous debate in the scientific community, but the case against using individual isolated calcium is strong, given that a meta-analysis, published in 2010 in the *British Medical Journal*, indicated that elemental (inorganic) calcium supplements increase the risk of cardiac infarction (heart attack).

Atherosclerosis

Calcium is a component of atherosclerotic plaque and when calcium salts build up in soft tissues it causes hardening, which is technically called calcification. Concerns regarding calcium supplementation have arisen because exposure to excess amounts of calcium over time sets the stage for endothelial dysfunction and formation of atherosclerotic plaque. However, this appears only to happen in the absence of adequate dietary magnesium.[8] The evidence for magnesium supplementation for bone health is already strong; see chapter 9 for further information on magnesium and its widespread health benefits. Professor Hansma also spoke about this subject in chapter 2, in relation to bone glue.

It is therefore surprising to see that most doctors are still prescribing inorganic calcium supplements, usually combined with vitamin D. These are certainly not the best option for bone-building available on the market, and it is unfortunate that they are prescribed against the growing body of evidence indicating that this approach gives little benefit for the reduction of fractures in the long term.

Chapter 7 summary

- Calcium is not as important to bone health as was previously thought.
- High calcium intake may not give protection from osteoporotic fractures.

- Large doses of inorganic calcium can interfere with the absorption of other minerals which are important for bone health.
- Inorganic calcium supplementation may increase the risk of heart attacks, and is therefore not recommended.
- Food-source calcium is far superior for bone health, and high-calcium green vegetables, such as kale, also contain many other beneficial bone-health minerals.

Chapter 8

Forgotten minerals

If, as we have just learned, calcium isn't as important for bone health as some of the other minerals, what are these others and where can we find them? Let's have a closer look at the many components of our bones and realise that they are so much more than just solidified lumps of chalk.

Magnesium

Could magnesium really be the mineral that 'does it all'? Although it is involved in over 50 biochemical reactions in the human body, it must be borne in mind that there are probably over 20,000 beneficial nutrients in plants and we need all of them. So no, there is no mineral, or vitamin, or antioxidant, or anything, for that matter, that is more important in the body than anything else that has also been shown to be essential for humans. However, because scientists like to isolate things from food and then test them on people, we have come to learn that a deficiency of certain nutrients can affect the body in a detrimental way.

Magnesium and bone strength

Magnesium is an element which is of vital importance for the human body, and is of particular relevance in bone strength, since 50 per cent of the body's magnesium is found in the bones.

Appropriate levels of magnesium are essential for adequate calcification of bone. Magnesium deficiency causes calcium crystals in the bone to have an abnormal shape, which negatively affects the resultant strength of the bone. Several steps in vitamin D metabolism, including its conversion to the 'supercharged' form that you will read about in chapter 9, depend on magnesium as a cofactor. In respect of bone health, it is already well known that vitamin D is an essential nutrient for bone strength and fracture resistance. It is currently proposed that magnesium deficiency could be an overlooked cause of low vitamin D status, adding yet more weight to the argument in favour of magnesium as an essential bone nutrient.[1]

One of the reasons why stress is so detrimental to bone health is that a surge in the adrenal hormone levels causes a large increase in urinary magnesium excretion – particularly problematic when it is estimated that large numbers of our population may be magnesium deficient in the first place. You'll find out more about stress and its harmful effects in chapter 11.

Eating your magnesium

The best food sources of magnesium are green leaves and green juices, particularly wheatgrass juice, if it is grown in highly mineralised soil. Anything with a high chlorophyll content will contain good levels of magnesium, since the central ion in the structure of chlorophyll is magnesium. Consider the different algae as well; they are excellent sources. Other good food sources include pumpkin seeds, artichokes, sprouted grains and buckwheat. We need to be aware of the concerns regarding magnesium depletion in the soil in which our food is grown. Some authors report that magnesium levels in farmland are too low in all countries except Egypt.

Processed food and magnesium status

One of the reasons that diets high in processed carbohydrates and refined sugar may negatively affect bone health is via their effect on bodily magnesium status. Refined sugar not only contains no magnesium, but it also causes the body to excrete magnesium through the kidneys. The process of producing refined sugar from sugar cane removes molasses, stripping the magnesium content entirely. Worse still, sugar does not simply reduce magnesium levels. Sweet foods are known by nutritionists as 'anti-nutrients'. Anti-nutrients are foods that replace whole nutritious foods in the diet, yet actually consume nutrients when digested, resulting in a net loss. Because all foods require vitamins and minerals to be consumed in order to power the process of digestion, it's important to choose foods that not only put back vital nutrients, but give a net gain. That is why a nutritionally dense plant-based diet is so important for the health of the bones, and of the whole body.

The more sweet foods and processed baked goods you have in your diet, the more likely you are deficient in magnesium and other vital nutrients.

Inaccuracies in testing

Testing for magnesium deficiency is potentially inaccurate. In a study published by the American College of Nutrition, it was noted that as many as 50 per cent of cases of magnesium deficiency are not recognised, due to statistical errors in the normal range set for serum (blood) magnesium testing.[2]

For those who have been shown to have, or are suspected of having, a low magnesium level, or are already on prescribed calcium tablets, supplementation with magnesium may be beneficial in the short to medium term; some researchers recommend longer periods of supplementation, for example up to a year, in those with a severe depletion. Indeed, Dr Carolyn Dean, author of *The Magnesium Miracle*, states that to obtain sufficient magnesium in the modern world, ongoing supplementation is essential, which it may be for those on a 'standard' Western diet. It is my opinion that when large daily salads and green juices become part of your lifestyle, you will be much less likely to suffer an ongoing magnesium deficiency, unless you are suffering from long-term depletion or chronic stress.

Magnesium spray

Much is currently being written in the alternative health world regarding the use of transdermal magnesium spray, also marketed as magnesium oil. This is potentially a very useful part of our anti-osteoporosis armoury, since we know that magnesium taken orally may be poorly absorbed, and also might cause diarrhoea. Those under chronic stress will often have low magnesium levels, and since stress is known to be a risk factor in osteoporosis, as discussed in more detail in chapter 11, transdermal magnesium spray could be a valuable method of replenishing the stores of this very important mineral.

In addition to poor bone strength, other health concerns relating to magnesium deficiency include diseases as varied as ADHD, chronic fatigue, atherosclerosis, stroke, hypertension, cramps, confusion and weakness. Since transdermal magnesium spray is well tolerated, perhaps it is something that everyone should consider as they age. Side effects associated with magnesium toxicity are very rare, but can occur in the presence of kidney failure. If you are concerned about using supplemental magnesium, check with your doctor first that your kidney function is normal; a simple blood and urine test will give you the information that you need regarding your kidneys.

Manganese

Its name sounds a bit like magnesium, doesn't it? It's not that similar, but it does play an important role in bone strength. Manganese works as a cofactor for several enzymes responsible for bone formation. It also stimulates the production of mucopolysaccharides (long chains of sugars which form complexes with proteins) in bone tissue, providing a structure upon which mineralisation can take place. Manganese deficiency results in abnormal skeletal development in a number of animal species. It is the preferred cofactor of enzymes called glycosyltransferases; these enzymes are required for the synthesis of large protein-sugar molecule combinations called proteoglycans, which are needed for the formation of healthy cartilage and bone. Impaired mucopolysaccharide formation as a result of manganese deficiency interferes with the process of bone calcification, and as a result, with remodelling, repair and ultimate formation of bone.[3]

Broken athletes and pollution

Manganese also came to light as being potentially important for bone health as a result of the investigation of some professional sportspeople who suffered from regular stress fractures. Their manganese levels were found to be very low, and once the deficiency was corrected, the stress fractures became a thing of the past.

Environmental pollutants such as cadmium interfere with our absorption of manganese, and food additives such as EDTA (ethylene diamine tetra-acetate) may inhibit its absorption. This is another good reason to be eating pure, organic, unadulterated food. Intensive farming practices deplete our soil of manganese. Calcium supplements prevent adequate absorption of manganese – another reason, as if we needed one, never to take individual isolated supplements, but to get our minerals from whole plants (with the possible exception of magnesium as discussed above). An optimal intake per day is not exactly known, but good sources of manganese are sprouted grains, sprouted chickpeas, nuts (in particular pine nuts), seeds and leafy green vegetables, particularly mustard greens and kale; all the staples used in a green vegetable-based, as opposed to fruit-based, living foods diet.

Other health benefits of manganese relate to the fact that it is present in the powerful antioxidant superoxide dismutase (SOD), the principal antioxidant used during energy production in the mitochondria.

Boron

OK, who's heard of boron? You may not have done, but it's probably at least as important as calcium when it comes to bone strength. Diets low in boron increase urinary excretion of both calcium and magnesium, a double whammy in favour of bone loss.[4] Increasing boron intake reverses this urinary excretion and boosts levels of 17-beta oestradiol and testosterone, two important hormones for bone health which are discussed later, in chapter 11.

Boron has many recognised effects in the body, and is involved in the enhancement of any processes involving hydroxylation, such as in the manufacturing of hormones. Hydroxylation sounds complicated, but it isn't too scary. It is basically a reaction in which an extra atom of both hydrogen and oxygen are added to a molecule, bringing about a change in the structure and function of that particular molecule. Boron is considered to enhance the conversion of vitamin D to its active form. You'll learn more about the importance of vitamin D later, in chapter 9.

Well-nourished soil leads to well-nourished people

The amount of boron in the diet depends ultimately on the amount available in the soil and water. Interestingly, in areas where boron in the water and soil is high, rates of arthritis appear to be low. Conversely, the bones of patients affected with arthritis show a much lower level of boron than healthy bones. Some studies indicate boron may help to protect against arthritis, or at least slow its progress by affecting the immune system's joint-damaging inflammatory response. Exactly how this happens is still unknown.

Boron enhances the effect of a variety of other nutrients, and works at the cell membrane aiding communications, entrances and exits of other better-known minerals. And while as yet no clear mechanism of action has emerged, that's no reason to ignore its importance.

The average Western diet provides about 1 mg of boron per day, but this can vary greatly. Many studies that have shown therapeutic or preventative effects of boron used about 3 mg per day. As always, do you need to rush out to buy the latest boron supplement? No; I think you might be able to guess what's coming next.

Boron is widely distributed in fruits, vegetables, nuts and legumes; apples are one of the better sources. A diet based on meat, eggs, dairy and cooked carbohydrates at the expense of fruits and vegetables is likely to be highly deficient in this important nutrient. Green leaves, cabbage, almonds, hazelnuts and apples are your best sources. Dandelion leaves are also high in boron, and additionally they are a good source of calcium, as well as silicon (see below). Scatter a few dandelion leaves in your salads; they are strong-tasting, but mixed with other greens you probably won't even notice them. Parsley is a good source of boron, so don't throw away that garnish of parsley on your plate. Parsley can be added to your green juice as well, and it is one of the ingredients in Juice Plus, a recommended food supplement (see Appendix 2).

It is stated that raisins are high in boron as well, but excessive dried fruit is contra-indicated for bone density due to the sugar content, so the recommendation is to get your boron from soaked almonds and plenty of greens.

Zinc

Better known as a mineral with benefits for men in relation to prostate health, zinc is found to be at low levels in the blood and bones of elderly people with osteoporosis.[5] Zinc enhances the biochemical actions of vitamin D (see chapter 9), and due to its role in DNA and protein synthesis, zinc is required for the formation of bone-building cells (osteoblasts) and formation of the proteins found in bone tissue. Zinc also inhibits the bone resorption caused by osteoclasts, the cells that break down old, worn-out bone that you read about in chapter 2.

Somewhat surprisingly, the food with the highest level of zinc is oysters; not exactly a plant-based food, and, according to Dr Brian Clement in his book *Killer Fish,* likely to be highly contaminated with toxic heavy metals such as mercury, as a result of widespread oceanic pollution. You won't therefore hear me recommending oyster consumption for the health of your bones, or any other body system for that matter. Soaked pumpkin seeds are your best plant-based source of zinc. Isolated supplementation with zinc is not something I recommend for osteoporosis reversal, since it interferes with levels of copper in the body – another mineral with important functions for bone strength, which is also discussed in this chapter.

Other health benefits of zinc

Zinc is important for the correct functioning of the immune system. The *European Journal of Immunology* states that zinc is essential for the activation of T-lymphocytes, which control and regulate immune functions, and attack infected and cancerous cells. Zinc deficiency can seriously impair immune functions,[6] but conversely zinc supplementation can reduce the duration of the common cold by up to 40 per cent.

Zinc also has benefits for memory and learning. Research conducted at the University of Toronto and published in the journal *Neuron* revealed that zinc has a crucial role in regulating how neurons communicate with one another, affecting how memories are formed and how we learn.

Zinc may play a part in the reduction of age-related macular degeneration (AMD), by reducing cellular damage in the retina. AMD can be prevented by ensuring the diet is high in the two specific antioxidants known to protect against retinal damage: lutein and zeaxanthin, found in green leaves and yellow vegetables, and in Juice Plus, a food supplement that I recommend to all my clients (see Appendix 2).

Strontium

Isn't strontium radioactive? Yes it can be, but that's strontium 90, which is present in nuclear fallout and has a half-life of over 28 years. Strontium 90 is not something you'd want to put in your body. The strontium we're talking about here is one of the most abundant elements on earth, which has an affinity for bone tissue. Strontium lies directly below calcium in group two of the periodic table, and shares many of its properties, so it's hardly surprising that it might play a role in bone strength. It has been demonstrated that strontium migrates to areas of bone where active remodelling is taking place, and rodent studies have shown that supplemental strontium led to increased bone density and formation. Small-scale studies have been performed on humans using isolated strontium with encouraging results in both osteoporosis and metastatic bone cancer.

A 2004 study from the *New England Journal of Medicine* suggests that strontium ranelate, a prescription medication, may be protective for women with osteoporosis. In a three-year study of postmenopausal women with osteoporosis, this form of strontium increased bone density in the hip and spine, and reduced the risk of vertebral fracture by 41 per cent compared to placebo. A longer-term study published by the same group in 2009 showed that strontium ranelate, compared to placebo, reduced the risk of vertebral fractures by 33 per cent over four years.

The forms of strontium found in supplements have not been subjected to testing in the same way that the prescription version has been. When taken at the recommended doses, strontium supplements appear to be safe, and side effects are rare, although they should be used with caution if there is a history of kidney disease or blood clots. Excessive doses of strontium may replace too much calcium in the bone and interfere with vitamin D metabolism, in turn causing the bones to weaken.

The optimal strontium dose is not known. If you are on medication treatment for osteoporosis, it is not known whether strontium supplements will enhance or diminish the benefits.

Also, it's important to note that whilst strontium may increase bone density, improvements seen on bone density testing may appear more impressive than they really are, just as with calcium. As stated previously, BMD does not exactly correlate with fracture risk.

Good soil is important

There is conflicting information regarding whether there is enough strontium present in food alone to be significant in the reversal of osteoporosis. As always, it depends what you read. Strontium levels in soil vary enormously around the globe and it all depends on where your food is grown. Growing your own food in enriched, organic soil is always the best option. Again, green leaves and sprouted grains are the best sources of this interesting mineral. Growing your own wheatgrass in mineral-rich soil and fertilising with diluted ocean water, as described by Maynard Murray in his book *Sea Energy Agriculture*, may well be an even better option, and will avoid any potential side effects that are often seen when one resorts to individual, isolated supplementation of one mineral whilst ignoring the others.

Other potential benefits of strontium

Other suggested benefits of strontium include its use as a treatment for metastatic bone cancer, and also for the possible reduction of dental cavities. Researchers are currently looking into its use for the relief of osteoarthritis, and a possibility that it might stimulate the regrowth of cartilage, following encouraging in vitro tests performed at the University of Liege, Belgium.

Copper

Copper is found in 13 enzyme systems, in particular those involved in forming strong bonds (cross-links). Copper is inhibited by excessive consumption of zinc, but this is usually only an issue in those taking isolated zinc supplements – yet another indication of why I do not recommend individual, isolated, non-food-derived supplements. Severe copper deficiency in growing children is known to cause bone abnormalities, so it is presumed that copper deficiency might be linked to osteoporosis. You probably won't be surprised to hear by now that by eating and juicing your greens, and taking wheatgrass juice, your copper levels will be sufficiently high to avoid putting yourself at risk. Sesame seeds and chick peas, staples of a good-quality plant-based diet, are rich sources of this mineral. Additional supplementation with isolated copper is not necessary unless you are supplementing with high doses of isolated zinc. The advice here of course would be not to take the zinc, or at least to be less enthusiastic with the dose.

Other health benefits of copper include its role in the antioxidant superoxide dismutase, and its involvement in the incorporation of iron into red blood cells, preventing anaemia. It is also involved in the generation of energy from carbohydrate metabolism inside the cells.

Silicon

There is a growing body of scientific literature which recognises that silicon has an essential role in bone formation and maintenance. Silicon improves bone matrix quality and facilitates bone mineralisation. Increased intake of bioavailable silicon has been associated with increased bone mineral density, and silicon supplementation in both animals and humans has been shown to increase bone mineral density and improve bone strength.[7] Interestingly, populations with the highest dietary intake of silicon (such as groups studied in India and China) have the lowest incidence of osteoporotic fractures.

The plant with the highest concentration of silicon is the horsetail, known to herbalists as Equisetum. The silicon in horsetail is in the form of monosilic acid, a form that the body can readily use. It is often used as a herbal tincture to promote bone strength, and not without good reason, since high concentrations of silicon are found at calcification sites of growing bone. Silicon is also involved in the formation of cartilage and other connective tissue. Silicon-deficient diets produced gross abnormalities of the bones of the skull in early experiments performed on animals many years ago.

In addition to horsetail, other good sources of silicon are cabbage, apples and whole grains. I recommend you to always use soaked and sprouted grains for the best bioavailability of nutrients and alkalinity, since as I mentioned earlier in chapter 4, heat-treated, hybridised grains are more likely to be acid forming, which will detract from bone health. For those people who are interested in a specific supplement, a product called BioSil is a liquid silicon extract containing monosilic acid. Six drops taken once daily with your green juice would give you enough silicon to help your bones and reverse any deficiency.

Cerveza, por favor?

Following on from some studies conducted in Spain in 2010, you might have heard that beer is being promoted as something we should drink for bone health, since beer apparently contains silicon (hops have been shown to have a high silicon content). However, since beer contains alcohol, it is to be avoided by the health seeker. I am unsure whether this study was funded by the alcoholic drinks industry; many such studies are. This practice has come to be known as 'chequebook science', whereby scientists are challenged to find something good in the product that is being promoted, such as beer, or wine, or cans of fizzy drink. Studies such as these regrettably do nothing to encourage people to change poor lifestyle habits, since the product being 'tested' ends up being portrayed in a more favourable light. This is one of the sad consequences of the food and drink industries and their massive budgets; it is only they who benefit, and not the end user.

Other reported benefits of increasing your silicon intake include strong nails, better skin quality and sleek, shiny hair, so the results are visible, provided that you are not trying to obtain your silicon from beer. You'll find out more about how alcohol damages your bones in chapter 10; you already know from chapter 4 that alcohol produces an undesirable acidic state in the body.

Germanium

No, not the garden plant (that's a geranium) – scour the internet for the mineral germanium and you will find it described as the 'miracle mineral' which will reverse cancer and solve all your health problems in one go. I always read such claims with a healthy dose of scepticism, but germanium has been shown to be valuable in increasing bone strength and reducing elevated levels of parathyroid hormone. It also helps with the detoxification of heavy metal elements that are known to be detrimental to bone strength, such as lead, cadmium and tin. Additionally it leads to oxygen enrichment of the tissues, which is important in its own right; particularly, as mentioned in chapter 2, for the correct functioning of osteocytes. However, there is always a downside, and overzealous use of isolated germanium supplementation can have serious side effects, such as kidney damage. As always, we want our minerals from food sources. So, where on earth can we find germanium? The mineral itself sounds very exotic, but you will be pleased to hear that a good source of germanium is good old garlic. Add it to your juice, salads or anything else you fancy; it really does do more than just boost your immune system.

Eat your greens

So is green best for your bones? All of the above minerals are found in abundance in greens, which leads to the development of strong bones, and, as you have seen, a host of other health benefits. To access these minerals you might have to do a bit of work, and for many a degree of lifestyle change will be essential. Probably the best way to access all those beneficial nutrients is by juicing. That way, any cellulose that was binding the minerals will be removed. Blending will also break down the cellulose, as will thorough chewing. Some authors disagree with eating raw greens and say that minerals are found in higher quantities in dark greens that have been boiled for an hour. I remain to be convinced by this. I don't agree that boiling could render anything more bioavailable than juicing would, and by boiling greens for that length of time, many of the heat-sensitive antioxidants and phytonutrients that have so many other health benefits would have long since been destroyed.

Chapter 8 summary

- There are numerous minerals other than calcium that are essential for bone health.
- Magnesium is essential for bone health and many people do not get enough of this mineral; supplementation is advisable, and the best form is an oil-based spray applied to the skin.
- Strontium, boron, zinc, copper, silicon and germanium are all important for bone health. These minerals are best obtained from whole, organically grown plant foods rather than via supplements.

Chapter 9

Overlooked vitamins and other phytonutrients

We all know that vitamins and other phytonutrients (also known as phytochemicals, the many thousands of extracts from plants that are beneficial to human health) are important for our health, but we tend to think that their benefits relate more to maintaining the health of the immune system and fighting free radical damage and ageing than building bone strength. Having looked at all the minerals that play a part in prevention and reversal of osteoporosis, and realising that there is so much more to it all than just calcium, perhaps it should not come as a great surprise that I now want to focus on the vitamins and other plant compounds that have been shown to have a vital role in healthy bone formation.

Vitamin C

Did I just type the wrong letter there? Surely many will have heard of the importance of vitamin D for bone health, but the effects of vitamin C are not as widely discussed. That's another reason for writing this book, since I wanted to point out the things that might be overlooked by the mainstream 'calcium and vitamin D' proponents. Vitamin C does indeed play a role in the strength of bone, by promoting the formation and cross-linking of some of its structural proteins, including collagen. In scurvy, which is a chronic vitamin C deficiency, various abnormalities are seen in the bones. Studies in guinea pigs, one of the few other mammals unable to manufacture their own vitamin C, indicate that a lack of this vitamin reduces the formation of, and increases the resorption (break down and dispersal of constituents) of, bone. Studies in postmenopausal women also indicate that the fracture rate is highest in those women with the lowest blood levels of vitamin C.[1]

As ever though, vitamin C is never the answer on its own, and if you are supplementing with vitamin C for other reasons, such as for cancer prevention, it is essential to use a whole-food supplement, not a synthetically derived one. And by following a high-greens raw diet, you will easily obtain enough of it from your food to avoid the need for additional supplementation. For all aspects of health, the section of the population with a higher than normal demand for vitamin C is the smokers, since smoking destroys this vitamin. Wholefood supplementation with additional vitamin C, not ascorbic acid, may be required until the habit is eliminated. My favourite wholefood supplement which provides excellent levels of bioavailable vitamin C, and has been clinically shown to boost blood levels of this important vitamin, is Juice Plus (see Resources and Appendix 2).

We probably don't need to be reminded about all the other health benefits of vitamin C – we've been hearing about them for years. According to an article in *Life Extension* magazine, published in 2008, one of the most interesting areas of study in relation to vitamin C is cardiovascular health. Researchers are finding that vitamin C impacts several aspects of cardiac health, ranging from blood pressure to endothelial health. Perhaps it's not surprising that as the relationship between oxidative damage, inflammation and atherosclerosis becomes increasingly investigated by science, vitamin C is seen as a key protective element against many aspects of cardiovascular disease.

However, it's important to never focus on just one antioxidant, since there are over 20,000 antioxidants present in fresh fruit and vegetables, and we need all of them in their natural form. Even in relation to heart disease, vitamin C is not necessarily the biggest player; that accolade could belong to resveratrol (see below), found in dark purple berries. As ever though, let's not be tempted to consider even this important antioxidant in isolation, exciting though it is to researchers. By removing resveratrol, and indeed vitamin C, from our food and taking it in isolation, we will not get the same benefits as we would from taking all of the phytonutrients that we find in a wide range of fruit and vegetables. Once again, this is why I only ever recommend taking supplements that are made from whole, unprocessed plants, and not synthetic isolates.

Vitamin K

Now here's a statement for you – vitamin K is as important for your bones as calcium. I have, however, never heard this statement from a doctor, or anyone else who is conducting bone density testing. No, calcium is all you will hear about. So how can vitamin K, which we tend to think of as being more important in the blood-clotting cascade than anything else, be beneficial for bones? It is firstly important to point out that there are different types of vitamin K, and the most commonly studied are K1, which is involved in blood clotting, and K2, which is important for bone health.

Biochemical cascade reactions are, to me at least, fascinating. Whilst studying A-level biology, and during my veterinary degree course, I came across numerous elegant and highly intricate pathways involved in everything from blood clotting to the production of energy. I was always fascinated to learn how these reactions worked, and how just one factor missing from a single stage of the sequence could mess everything else up. Vitamin K2 could indeed be one such factor, especially when we consider that it is required for the production of osteocalcin, one of the structural proteins in bone: a protein which is the matrix upon which bone mineralisation occurs. Osteocalcin provides order and structure to bone tissue and the action of vitamin K allows it to attract calcium ions. Vitamin K2 therefore plays a very important role – without it the bones would be much more like chalk – fragile and very easily broken.

Do we get enough?

For the most part, we have been taught that general vitamin K deficiency is extremely rare, and therefore it has not been greatly studied in relation to bone density. Information is emerging now that indicates these preliminary assumptions could be incorrect, and elderly people have been highlighted as a population group whose vitamin K levels might be lower than optimal.

Animal studies have shown that a diet low in vitamin K increases urinary calcium excretion, which is reversed when vitamin K is added back to the diet. Of the studies that have been conducted, vitamin K2 has been demonstrated to stimulate bone formation via the action of osteoblasts, our bone-building cells, and to inhibit the resorption of bone by osteoclasts, the cells that break down bone.[2] Other studies indicate that the use of vitamin K2 caused significantly increased levels of osteocalcin, a biomarker of bone formation. Additionally, vitamin K2 was shown also to inhibit a reduction in bone calcium content by blocking bone-resorbing factors such as parathyroid hormone.

Vitamin K2 provides two critical benefits to the bones. Firstly, it protects against excess bone degradation by turning off excess osteoclast activity. Secondly, it supports the critical role of new bone formation by enabling osteocalcin to pull calcium from the blood and layer it on to the bone.

No vitamin is an island

You probably won't be surprised to learn that vitamin K does not act alone in its involvement in bone building. We already know that maintenance of healthy bone tissue requires adequate levels of minerals, vitamin D and vitamin K. Without vitamin D (see below), there would be no osteocalcin for vitamin K to work on. Without vitamin K, the osteocalcin that is produced would be inactive. Without calcium and the other minerals discussed in the previous chapter, there would be no minerals for the activated osteocalcin to attract to the bone for structural density. Isn't it fascinating how all these things work together? I'm sure you can now see why I don't agree with those who only recommend calcium and vitamin D supplements for bone building.

The *Nurses' Health Study* followed more than 72,000 women for 10 years, and found that women whose vitamin K intakes were in the lowest quintile (1/5) had a 30 per cent higher risk of hip fracture than women with vitamin K intakes in the highest four quintiles.[3]

Despite encouraging findings such as these, conflicting studies exist on the importance of vitamin K2 to bone health. Indeed, some authors state that although observational studies have shown correlations between vitamin K intake and lower risk of fractures in older adults, the current evidence from randomised controlled trials is surprisingly not sufficiently supportive of vitamin K supplementation for the intent of improving bone health.

Can we make it?

Vitamin K1 is converted to K2 in various organs of the body, although it is argued that this process is potentially inefficient, and even those with a high vitamin K1 intake from food could potentially have lower than optimal levels of K2. The form of vitamin K2 most generally recognised to play an important role in bone health is menaquinone. Some authors insist that humans do not easily convert K1 to K2; therefore animal products should be eaten to ensure that K2 levels are adequate. However, the best dietary source of menaquinone is natto, a fermented soya product, so it is not actually necessary to consume animal products to obtain K2, even if your conversion pathway is less than adequate.

The best source of vitamin K1, once again, is dark green leafy vegetables. However, another problem faces us, and that is that we may be inadvertently reducing our body's vitamin K levels in another way. Much of the vitamin K2 present in the body is produced by the intestinal microflora – our 'friendly bacteria'. The widespread usage of antibiotics in modern medicine, particularly broad spectrum antibiotics, wipes out these beneficial microbes and therefore reduces our supply of vitamin K2, no matter what we are eating. A sensible approach therefore in the reversal of osteoporosis might be to restore probiotic levels, so that we can naturally boost our vitamin K levels, as well as eating all those greens.

Maintaining healthy levels of probiotics seems to extend beyond vitamin K. Preliminary small-scale experiments in rats and humans have indicated that feeding a supplement of galacto-oligosaccharides (a pre-biotic fibre) which acts as 'food' for our probiotics, increase not only the absorption and bone retention of calcium and magnesium, but also increase the BMD of the femur (thigh bone) and tibia (shin) in the rat model, and make the bone more resistant to fracture. It has therefore been concluded that our friendly bacteria have an important role to play in bone health.[4]

Further difficulties relating to the absorption of vitamin K are also encountered if people have low gastric hydrochloric acid levels. I discuss this phenomenon in considerable detail in *The Whole Body Solution*. Suffice it to say here that inadequate levels of hydrochloric acid in the stomach interfere with the absorption of many nutrients, including calcium, vitamin B12, vitamin C and iron.

Warfarin and vitamin K

A word of caution in relation to vitamin K for those people on anticoagulants: if you are taking anticoagulants such as warfarin, discuss your dosage of these drugs with your doctor if you want to radically change your diet to incorporate a lot of vitamin K-rich foods. Alternatively, and as recommended by *Life Extension* magazine, ask if you can supplement with a small amount of vitamin K2, which will often stabilise INR readings (the measurement by which therapeutic levels of the anticoagulant warfarin are assessed). A final option to discuss with your doctor would be changing from warfarin to heparin; heparin is a different type of anticoagulant which does not involve the vitamin K pathways, but may have other side effects, so be sure that you are well informed prior to making any decisions about changes in medication.

Other health benefits of vitamin K2

One of the most interesting findings with regard to vitamin K2 supplementation relates to the rate of calcification in the body, notably that of the arteries. Calcification of the arteries is a very undesirable situation, which adversely affects the whole cardiovascular system, often with devastating consequences. Vitamin K2 seems to reduce the likelihood of arterial calcification by ensuring that calcium stays in the bones, rather than being deposited in the soft tissues of the body. Many age-related diseases can be linked to calcification, including kidney stones, arthritis, cataracts, heart valve insufficiency, wrinkled skin, bone spurs, senility and, as already mentioned, atherosclerosis. It is suggested that restoring optimal vitamin K2 levels might help to protect against such disorders.

Folic acid

One of the B-vitamins, folic acid is better known for its role in pregnancy in reducing the occurrence of neural tube defects and protection against spina bifida. However, it does additionally have rather important benefits for our bones, via another of those fascinating biochemical pathways.

Homocysteine dangers: hearts and bones

One of the compounds that is now being regularly measured as a useful indicator for the development of heart disease is homocysteine. Homocysteine is a compound that is produced from the metabolism of methionine, an amino acid. Methionine is present in much higher levels in meat, chicken, fish and eggs than in plant proteins, and the more methionine we ingest, the higher our homocysteine levels can become, unless we have adequate folic acid to counteract the problem. High homocysteine is a risk factor not only for heart disease, but, it would appear, also for osteoporosis. Those afflicted with the genetic condition homocysteinuria, in which abnormally high homocysteine levels appear in both the blood and the urine, often develop atherosclerosis and osteoporosis by the age of 20. Additional studies are putting homocysteine forward as another possible biomarker for fracture risk.[5]

The onset of menopause brings a reduced ability to detoxify homocysteine, and this in turn is one of the factors involved in the rapid increase in the incidence of both heart disease and osteoporosis in postmenopausal women. Studies in Sweden have shown that supplementing with additional folic acid, even in those subjects whose blood levels of folic acid were considered to be normal, significantly reduced the levels of homocysteine in the blood; 5 mg of folic acid per day was found to reduce plasma homocysteine levels by over 50 per cent in just 14 days.

The mechanisms by which homocysteine metabolism becomes less efficient after menopause are not fully understood. It is also not known whether a level of folic acid as high as 5 mg per day, as in the aforementioned study, is really necessary.

I would caution against isolated doses this high, or even perhaps doses greater than 1 mg, since folic acid can interfere with zinc absorption, and if used for weeks to months, may mask vitamin B12 deficiency, and even produce damaging folacin crystals in the kidneys. However, what has been demonstrated, and I will discuss this further in the section on supplementation, is that there is a wholefood-based supplement that has been shown to build bone strength, even in the absence of exercise, which also slashes homocysteine levels. That product is Juice Plus, and I view this as very useful in our armoury against osteoporosis.

Once again, the best source of folic acid is ... fresh raw vegetables, so eat (and juice) your greens.

Vitamin B6

Vitamin B6 is important in bone strength since it also, along with folic acid, plays a part in the metabolism of homocysteine. There is a suspected widespread deficiency of B6 in the Western world due to the presence of antimetabolites to B6; substances which interfere with its function. Hydrazines, a type of industrial chemical, and food colourings, herbicides and plant growth regulators are all likely to interfere with the proper functioning of vitamin B6. The usefulness of this vitamin is not confined to its action in homocysteine metabolism. It is also a cofactor for the enzyme lysyl oxidase, which cross-links structural proteins and connective tissue, giving tensile strength to bone. It is also involved in the production of progesterone, an essential hormone for bone strength, which is discussed in the hormones section in chapter 11.

Excessive supplementation with vitamin B6 has been linked to neurological damage and severe impairment of sensory nerve function, underlining, yet again, the fact that vitamins should never be taken individually in high doses. The best sources always come from wholefood. In the case of vitamin B6, good levels are found in bananas, red peppers, spinach, sprouted chick peas, sweet potato and sprouted grains.

Finally, another reason why smokers are more prone to osteoporosis may well be that they are often deficient in vitamin B6 as a result of the hydrazine present in cigarette smoke.

Resveratrol

Resveratrol is an interesting antioxidant which has recently been catapulted to almost superstar status on the natural health radar. Similar to the flurry of scientific interest generated by vitamin C all those years ago when it was first discovered, resveratrol is the new superhero of the nutritional researcher, and it has exploded onto the health scene, with followers taking it in huge amounts in the hope that it is going to be the answer to their supplement prayers and protect them from all known ills. In addition to its known benefits for cardiovascular health, researchers are now indicating that it could be useful in the reversal of osteoporosis, following a study conducted by French researchers in 'weightless' rats, in which space flight, and the muscle wastage that occurs in such trips, was mimicked. A daily dose of resveratrol given to the rats prevented bone and muscle wastage,[6] so it is now hypothesised that similar findings might be anticipated in sedentary humans.

Inflammation

Resveratrol is known to affect genes that modulate the inflammatory process, and it has been shown that people with high inflammatory biomarkers have an imbalance of osteoblasts to osteoclasts, tipping the balance away from bone building and towards bone breakdown. By influencing this process, and positively affecting genes that encourage bone building, resveratrol may have beneficial effects on skeletal health in the long term. Whilst the marketers of red wine will no doubt want you to know that resveratrol is the antioxidant that makes red wine 'healthy', please do not be misled into thinking that drinking red wine will enhance your bone health; it will not. And please also be aware that it is not just the skins of dark grapes that contain resveratrol; high levels are found in blueberries, blackberries and all the other blue / black / purple berries that exist.

Brilliant blueberries

Two particularly interesting studies relating to bone health have been conducted on rats which were fed blueberries, in experiments that mimicked both early life and later life. The first, involving young rats, indicated that those fed the blueberries had a range of phenolic acids (of which resveratrol is one type) in the blood, which appeared to significantly stimulate the differentiation of osteoblasts, resulting in significantly increased bone mass.[7] This is an exciting finding since it indicates that blueberries, a low-glycaemic, low-sugar-content berry, could provide a way in which to increase peak bone mass and delay degenerative bone disorders such as osteoporosis. It was also a 'dietary induced' study; the rats were fed the blueberries, rather than being injected with a chemical compound, which indicates that the blood levels of the beneficial compounds were rising just in response to eating food.

The second study involved ovariectomised rats; those whose ovaries had been removed, which provides a model for women after menopause. The findings of this study indicated that blueberries can prevent bone loss as seen not just by increased bone mineral density, but also by favourable changes in biomarkers of bone metabolism.[8]

Other health benefits of resveratrol

Many other health benefits have been attributed to resveratrol, ranging from enhanced muscular endurance (useful for long distance athletes), improved cardiovascular health as a result of reductions in atherosclerotic plaque, reduction in the likelihood of colon cancer and improved blood flow to the brain, enhancing mental agility. One study in mice even indicated that it can be responsible for boosting testosterone levels; important in its own right, since, as you'll read in chapter 11, testosterone is a hormone with positive effects on bone health and reduction in fractures.

Despite all the many health benefits attributed to resveratrol, please be aware that, as with all other antioxidants, it does not act in isolation. It is the synergy of all the antioxidants acting together which give the best benefits for bodily health, not the process of extracting a single antioxidant, concentrating it, putting it into a pill and expecting it to do the same thing. That is why, when looking for a food supplement that contains all the nutrients (known and unknown) that we need for good health, it's so important to only use those which are made from whole plants. Those which might have initially been extracted from plants, but have subsequently been artificially concentrated into mega-doses of only one or two nutrients (such as resveratrol on its own) will no longer be in synergy and the benefits will not be the same. By concentrating individual nutrients in this way, nature's subtle orchestration is lost, and the risks of side effects or overdosage become more likely. More of one nutrient, taken in isolation, is not better. See Appendix 2 for information on the supplement that I personally use, which contains not just blueberries but six other beneficial berries and a total of 17 other foods with proven benefits for human health.

Curcumin (from turmeric root)

Curcumin is one of the active phytonutrients in turmeric root, a member of the ginger family. It is another phenolic compound, like resveratrol, and has been used in the Ayurvedic health system for thousands of years. Approximately 2,600 research papers have been published recognising the potential health benefits of the curcuminoids present in turmeric root, with most of the more important studies having been published within the last two decades.

Considering cytokines

To consider how curcumin might be effective, we first need to meet some molecules called cytokines. Cytokines are small proteins released by cells, several of which trigger undesirable inflammation in the body. The 'code' for production of these inflammatory cytokines is embedded in our DNA. However, as it transpires, we don't have to activate their production; indeed, we can suppress it. The molecule responsible for telling our DNA to produce these cytokines is NF-κB, or 'nuclear factor-kappaB' to give it its full name.

Via production of these cytokines, NF-κB is considered to be responsible for harmful levels of inflammation in the body, and responsible in part for many disease processes. Therefore blocking this effect, by suppressing NF-κB, is proving to be beneficial, and, luckily for us, turmeric consumption is one of the ways in which this can be achieved.[9] This is important to bone health since the activation of NF-κB has been linked to osteoporosis, as well as disease processes as diverse as cancer, atherosclerosis, diabetes, allergies, asthma, arthritis, Crohn's disease, MS, Alzheimer's disease, septic shock and AIDS.

Affecting osteoclasts

The way in which suppression of NF-κB is thought to be beneficial for bone health is that it slows down the process via which osteoclasts are produced. In chapter 2, we learned that osteoclasts are the cells which break down old, worn-out bone.

By slowing down the rate of development of young, inactive osteoclasts into adult, active osteoclasts, the process of bone breakdown is also slowed. Some prescription drugs are now available which block this process completely (they are called RANK-Ligand inhibitors, discussed in chapter 10), but do bear in mind that osteoclasts are actually necessary; they get rid of old bone that has outlived its usefulness, and prevent the bones from becoming too thick and bulky.

In effect, everyone can benefit from the addition of fresh, or even dried, turmeric root to the diet, and the great news is that it has no adverse side effects. I recommend using the fresh root in green juices and soups, and the dried turmeric powder as a condiment in any dish. Ginger root is also being found to possess similar properties as a result of a phytonutrient called 6-gingerol – a natural analogue of curcumin which exhibits a biological activity similar to that of curcumin.[10]

Vitamin D

Sunny side up! This is the vitamin we have all heard of in relation to strong bones, and it has been somewhat misnamed, since vitamin D is actually a hormone, made from cholesterol. Vitamin D is formed in the skin upon exposure to ultraviolet light (UVB rays), so sun exposure is very important in the quest to prevent osteoporosis.

Sunny pathways

The vitamin D made in our skin on exposure to the UVB rays then travels to the liver, where it is converted to a vitamin D metabolite, whose function is to act as the 'storage' form of vitamin D (stored in both the liver and fat cells). When vitamin D is needed, some of the stored form is transported to the kidneys, where an enzymatic reaction converts it to what T. Colin Campbell, author of *The China Study*, describes as 'supercharged' vitamin D (also known as 1,25

D or 25 (OH)D), which is approximately 1000 times more active than the storage form. Yet another concern regarding diets high in animal protein is that they cause a decrease in levels of 1,25 D; the acidic environment that animal protein causes blocks the kidney enzyme from producing this supercharged metabolite.[11] Likewise, those with high stress levels might be inadvertently affecting their vitamin D levels; high levels of cortisol adversely affect vitamin D absorption, in addition to being damaging to the process of bone formation itself.

Sun fears

There exists considerable controversy about sun exposure. How many times have we heard that we have to wear at least factor 15 sunblock before we consider venturing outside, even in the UK in winter? This was recently taken to extremes by a lady in Southampton, the city closest to my home, who used so much sunblock on her 12-year-old daughter that the unfortunate child developed rickets as a result. In contrast, I was always out in the sun as a child, without any sunblock. My mother regularly checked how long I had been outside and made me come inside, or put more clothes on me, to prevent my skin from burning. We seem to have become so consumed with the fear of malignant melanoma, the most dangerous form of skin cancer, that many of us get insufficient sun exposure to stimulate adequate vitamin D production. Vitamin D deficiency is becoming rife in our society, and it has been linked to numerous other medical problems; unsurprisingly perhaps, when we consider that vitamin D receptors have been found in as many as 300 locations in the human body.

The vitamin D/calcium connection

Vitamin D is essential for calcium and phosphorus absorption in the gut and its deposition into the bones. 1,25 D controls the levels of calcium in the blood and keeps it within its optimal range, together with the action of parathyroid hormone. If calcium consumption is too high (such as with overuse of chalk-based supplements) it lowers the activity of the kidney converting enzyme, and the levels of 1,25 D fall, indicating that high calcium diets are not necessarily better for us.[12] It is estimated that half the population of the UK is deficient in vitamin D in the winter, with as many as one in six being classified as severely deficient. Those more at risk are the dark skinned who live too far away from the equator, women who use a traditional religious dress which prevents any exposure of their skin to the sun, and anyone who lives at latitudes greater than 40 degrees north or south of the equator. Additionally, those living in a polluted environment will have less exposure to UVB, since air pollution blocks some of the UVB rays reaching us. Older people also seem to have a lower rate of production of vitamin D in the skin when exposed to sunlight; by the age of 70, their ability to produce vitamin D in the skin is considered to be reduced by 75 per cent in comparison with people aged 20.

Food or sun?

According to the Vitamin D Council, food sources of vitamin D are of lesser significance here since 90 per cent of our vitamin D supplies come from sun exposure, not food. However, certain mushrooms have been shown to have relatively good levels and are used in supplementation regimes. In northern Europe the humble stinging nettle gives a good supply, so put some gloves on and pick some fresh nettles to go in your daily green juice. You may hear that the only food source of vitamin D is from animal products. This is not actually the case – we just have to be a bit more resourceful in where we look. Nettles are also a good source of vitamin K, which has been discussed on page 85.

An interesting study conducted by Dr Luigi Fontana et al from

Washington University School of Medicine (St. Louis) indicated that people following a living-foods, uncooked plant-based diet absorbed and maintained higher levels of vitamin D than the many others tested on a multitude of different diets. The body mass index (BMI) of these subjects, and their bone density as measured by DEXA scanning, was lower on average than those following other diets, but the researchers did not equate this apparently low bone mass to an increased fracture risk, since other biomarkers of bone health were normal.[13] There is good reason, and it is not by accident that, in the recipe section at the back of this book, I have included a variety of recipes which follow these dietary principles. Retaining good levels of vitamin D is vital to bone health, and the more methods by which we can enhance our levels, the better.

The vitamin D/vitamin K connection

I recommend that anyone concerned about their vitamin D levels, and whether they should be supplementing, get tested for 1,25 D. Despite recommendations from the Vitamin D Council that it is safe to take up to 10,000 IU (international units) per day, I advise against indiscriminate supplementation with vitamin D, particularly if you have regular sun exposure, since high serum levels are now being linked with an increased risk of pancreatic cancer.[14] Remember also that the signs of vitamin D toxicity are just as likely to be vitamin K2 deficiency. When you take vitamin D, the body creates more vitamin K2-dependent proteins that move calcium around in the body. Without vitamin K2, those proteins remain inactivated, so their benefits are unrealised. This is why, when supplementing, I recommend supplements that contain 1,25 D and K2 together, for the best health benefits. Taken together, these two nutrients keep the calcium in your bones and improve heart health by preventing the arteries and other soft tissues from becoming calcified.

How much sun?

For those concerned about adequate sun exposure with minimal associated risk, my recommendations are to use some common sense. Do not go out in the sun at midday at the equator and stay there for three hours; build up gradually. After a long winter, expose slowly, for a few minutes a day, if you have very pale skin. Avoid the sun between 11am and 3pm as a general rule. But do expose! I have friends who deliberately travel to the tropics or southern hemisphere to avoid the British winter, for the main purpose of boosting their vitamin D levels. I hope to join them there one day.

Regarding sunblock, avoid chemical sunblocks, since the skin will absorb practically everything you put onto it. Standard sunblock is full of many undesirable chemicals, which some authors postulate may even be linked to the development of melanomas – the very thing that people are using the sunblock to prevent. Personally I never use sunblock unless I am up a mountain (altitude increases your 'dose' of UVB rays), and I am well known for my love of being out in the sun. My favourite form of protection is close-woven cotton clothes, as recommended by the Vitamin D Council.

A final word of warning regarding sun exposure supplying you with adequate vitamin D is that if you shower within 12 hours of the sun exposure, you wash off the oils in the skin that are being converted. New studies even indicate that it could be up to 48 hours before the vitamin D has been absorbed, and most people would certainly have showered by then. The advice therefore would be to go out in the sun early in the day, and not shower until the following morning.

Other benefits of vitamin D

Multiple sclerosis

The main reported concern regarding vitamin D deficiency in the health and scientific literature is that of the increased incidence of multiple sclerosis (MS) in the presence of low vitamin D levels. MS is well known to be more prevalent in those who live further away from the equator, and also in those who consume more dairy products. For example, the incidence of MS in the south of Australia is reported to be seven times that in the north of the country.[15] Those with the lowest vitamin D status have more severe disability. Vitamin D plays a part in MS as a result of its action on Th1 cells: a type of T cell in the adaptive immune system. Th1 cells attack the myelin sheath (fatty insulation) of the nerve fibres, causing the nerve-damaging effects that are classically seen with MS. Vitamin D regulates and modifies the potentially self-destructive actions of these Th1 cells, reducing the damage to the nerves. People exposed to the sun when young seem to have less likelihood of developing MS when older.

Cancer

Whilst some authors report that the benefits of higher blood vitamin D levels bring a reduction in the risk of certain cancers, for example colorectal cancer, others have found no, or weak, correlations. I mentioned IGF-1 in chapter 3 in regard to dairy products, and the fact that enhanced production of IGF-1 enhances the growth of cancer cells. When blood levels of 1,25 D are low, IGF-1 becomes more active, increasing the production of new cells and inhibiting the destruction of old. This is of significant concern, since people with higher than normal IGF-1 levels in their blood have been shown to have a more than five times greater risk of advanced-stage prostate cancer.[16] Animal-based foods such as meat and dairy lead to more IGF-1 and less 1,25 D, both of which increase cancer risk.

Other studies have indicated benefits of vitamin D supplementation in the reduction of breast cancer. A Creighton University study showed that women over the age of 55 who took a 1,100 IU per day vitamin D supplement, with calcium, and were followed for four years had a highly statistically significant ($P<0.005$) 75 per cent reduction in breast cancer, diagnosed after the first 12 months, compared with women who took a placebo.[17] Additionally, Dr Cedric Garland, professor of family and preventive medicine at the University of California, has stated: 'We found that daily intakes of vitamin D by adults in the range of 4,000 to 8,000 IU are needed to maintain blood levels of vitamin D metabolites in the range needed to reduce by about half the risk of several diseases, including breast cancer.' He even went as far as to make the bold statement that, in his opinion, breast cancer could be virtually eradicated by raising vitamin D levels.

Autoimmune diseases

Information from the Vitamin D Council indicates that certain autoimmune diseases, such as systemic lupus erythematosus, are more prevalent in people whose vitamin D levels are low. Anecdotal evidence exists that lupus flares are less acute and can be controlled with vitamin D supplementation.

DNA repair and metabolic processes

Dr Michael Holick, author of *The Vitamin D Solution*, conducted a study on healthy volunteers taking 2,000 IU of vitamin D per day for a few months. His findings were that the participants upregulated 291 different genes that control up to 80 different metabolic processes: from improving DNA repair to having an effect on autoxidation (oxidation that occurs in the presence of oxygen and/or ultraviolet radiation, which has implications for ageing and cancer, for example), boosting the immune system, and many other biological processes.

Whilst it is true that whole books have been written on the importance of vitamin D, please be aware that it is no more, and no less, important for bone and whole-body health than all the other nutrients and lifestyle factors that are discussed in this book. Please ensure that you pay attention to all of them; your bones, and in turn your whole body, will love you for it.

Chapter 9 summary

- Low levels of vitamin C are associated with higher fracture rates, so fresh vegetables with good vitamin C content are essential for bone health.
- Vitamin K is essential for bone health, and many people may be deficient in vitamin K, or lack the ability to absorb and utilise it adequately.
- Boosting gut probiotic levels is important for bone health.
- Adequate intake of the B vitamins B6 and folic acid are essential for bone strength.
- Nutrients found in dark-skinned berries and turmeric are important for our overall health, including that of our bones.
- Vitamin D deficiency strongly correlates with poor bone health. Inadequate exposure to sunlight adversely affects our bone strength and is increasingly being linked to many other diseases, including cancer and multiple sclerosis.
- All of the nutrients discussed here, with the possible exception of vitamin D, can be found in fruits, vegetables, nuts, seeds and legumes. Basing your diet around these food choices is your best ally for bone-building success.

Chapter 10

Supplements and drugs – the good, the bad and the downright ugly

I must have lost count of the number of supplements I have seen that have been specifically targeted towards those concerned about their bone density, which contain only inorganic calcium (i.e. chalk!) and magnesium, if we're lucky, and nothing else. With all the information that has been presented so far, surely we know that we should now be avoiding such things, or at least starting to demand from the manufacturers details of clinical trials that show that their product has a positive impact on the achievement of either increased bone density, or reduction in fractures, or preferably both. In nearly all of these cases, no such research exists. These unscrupulous manufacturers are playing on the consumers' lack of knowledge of the importance of elements other than calcium, and profiting from the sale of supplements that have absolutely no clinical value. Caveat emptor: let the buyer beware.

The most important questions to ask regarding any kind of supplementation you are offered, or recommended to use, in relation to osteoporosis or indeed anything else, are as follows:

1. How has the supplement been produced? This is of vital importance. If it has been synthetically prepared from individual, isolated ingredients, rather than being extracted from whole plants, it will be of very limited, if

any, value, and potentially be harmful, as we have seen in the case of calcium.

2. How has the supplement been processed? If it is made from whole plants, but has been processed at high temperatures, the heat-labile factors such as all the vitamins we have just been discussing will have been denatured, and therefore will be of limited or no value.
3. Is the supplement bioavailable? In other words, when you take it, has it been demonstrated to get into the blood stream or the organs in which it is needed? If bioavailability studies have been performed, where are they published? Have they, for example, been published in a peer-reviewed scientific journal?
4. Has the research been performed on this particular supplement, or has it, for example, been performed on an ingredient which is present in the supplement, and therefore it is only assumed that the supplement in question will have the same effect?
5. Are there any adverse side effects known from the use of this supplement? If so, where are the results published? If the person you are asking starts to squirm and starts looking uncomfortable, you can pretty much guarantee that their supplement has no research backing it that would give validity to its use. We are not, after all, designed to lick rocks to get our minerals. We need to eat food that was grown in highly mineralised soil. Plants can take up minerals from soil into their structure. Humans cannot.

So, should we be using food supplementation for prevention and reversal of osteoporosis? Absolutely, yes, in my opinion. Let's think back to the previous sections and consider what we have learned.

Chapter 10

The good

Algae

We have discovered in chapter 4 how acidity can greatly influence bone loss. Therefore my first recommendation for food supplementation is liquid blue-green algae (commercially available as a supplement called E3Live). It is one of the most alkalising foods on the planet and if taken daily with green juices it will aid in the reduction of bone mineral loss due to excessive acidity. E3Live has many other benefits, being very high in all the alkaline minerals, and containing excellent levels of all the important vitamins that we need for bone health. I am not aware of any specific studies performed on it in relation to reduction in hip fractures, but its broad nutritional spectrum and nutrient bioavailability make it an excellent choice for overall health of many body tissues, including bone. One scientific study has indicated a potential benefit of spirulina, a type of blue-green algae, for its anti-osteoporotic effects on rats treated with an anti-diabetic drug,[1] so it could also give potential benefits for humans, and has no adverse side effects.

Wheatgrass juice

Wheatgrass is really a food rather than a supplement, and contains one of the broadest spectra of bioavailable minerals, particularly if grown with the use of *Ocean Solution* (diluted ocean water), or in mineral-enriched soil. It is an essential part of the health seeker's diet. Dried powdered wheatgrass will not have the same benefits, since it is generally made from the whole leaf of the plant, which still contains cellulose, which in turn might affect the bioavailability of the supplement. Wheatgrass needs to be used freshly juiced for best effects. It has been one of the staples at the Hippocrates Health Institute for over 50 years. It is also alkalising, so reduces the urinary mineral loss we see that is associated with excess tissue acidity, as well as replenishing the body with essential minerals. In fact, it contains 102 different vitamins and minerals. For more information on the benefits of wheatgrass juice, please see my website www.therawfoodscientist.com.

Wholefood-derived supplements

The importance of using vitamins and minerals from wholefood sources cannot be overstated. As we have seen in chapter 8, an excess of one mineral can lead to a deficiency in others, and many minerals are also toxic at high doses. It therefore makes no sense to try to outsmart nature, by taking individual isolated supplements of any vitamin or mineral, inevitably guessing the quantity that might be needed. We really have moved on from that approach, and 95 per cent of vitamin and mineral supplements sold in stores have absolutely no validity for their use. Interestingly, many of them are made by the pharmaceutical industry.

I am pleased, therefore, to mention something I feel is worthy of your consideration – Juice Plus. I have personally used this wholefood supplement for 20 years. Why? Because it is wholefood-based and processed at low temperatures, so that the enzymes remain intact, satisfying questions one and two above. It is bioavailable, and has published studies to support that claim. It has been scientifically demonstrated to lower homocysteine levels, one of the risk factors for osteoporosis and heart disease which has already been discussed. Additionally it has been scientifically proven in several published studies to elevate the levels of important vitamins and minerals which we know are necessary for osteoporosis prevention. This is not surprising, since it contains a good number of the foods known to be high in these beneficial minerals and vitamins. This is encouraging stuff so far. But most importantly in this context is that there is also a study (as yet unpublished) indicating that it was able to increase bone density in test subjects who did not change their diet or exercise regime. For more information, please see www.juiceplus.co.uk/+mt016459, which is my specific website for this product, and see the studies listed in Appendix 2.

Bioidentical hormone replacement

Bioidentical hormones are receiving a lot of press right now in the health world, and I will discuss their use more fully in the next chapter. They can be considered to be good things to use, but blood tests must always be carried out first to ascertain blood levels of the six sex hormones that play a role in our health, including our bone strength, as we age. Indiscriminate usage of even nature-identical hormones can have serious consequences if we don't know what we're doing.

Wholefood calcium

Plant sources of calcium are also receiving a lot of attention. By now you will of course realise that calcium is only a small part of the jigsaw that is bone health, but if you want to take a supplement that is a good source of calcium, which also contains balanced levels of magnesium, please make sure that the only one you use is this one – Bone Support, from Nature's Plus, as recommended earlier. It is made from a whole plant that is known to be rich in calcium, and also contains a large number of the other beneficial nutrients, including vitamins D and K2, that have been discussed above. Because the nutrients in this supplement come from plants, the body will know what to do with them. The nutrients will be recognised as food, rather than an indigestible lump of rock, which is in fact what practically all other mineral supplements on the market are.

Vitamin D

If you have been found to be deficient in 1,25 D on a blood test, the best oral supplement I have come across thus far is made by the Hippocrates Health Institute. It is called *Sun D*, and is made from mushrooms. For Hippocrates' online store, visit www.hippocratesinst.org. For those wishing to place orders in the UK, visit www.fresh-network.com.

Probiotics

I mentioned in chapter 9 that vitamin K is depleted in individuals who have received long-term, or broad-spectrum, antibiotic treatment, because the friendly microorganisms in the gut are responsible in part for maintaining good levels of vitamin K. Therefore if you have used antibiotics frequently, either in the past or recently, a decent course of a good-quality, broad-spectrum probiotic is definitely advantageous. My preferred brand is Nature's Biotics, available in the UK from Kiki Health (www.kiki-health.com).

Digestive enzymes

Finally, as we age, it is well known that our digestive systems become less efficient, therefore reducing our ability to absorb the nutrients we need from our food. Elderly people who have already been diagnosed with osteoporosis, and anyone who wishes to extract the maximum benefit from all the good food they are eating, would be well advised to take digestive enzymes, and have a test to check that their levels of hydrochloric acid are not too low, as I discuss in my book *The Whole Body Solution*. For enzyme supplementation, *HHI-Zyme*, the Hippocrates Institute's product, is the one I recommend to use. It can be obtained via the Hippocrates online store and via Kiki Health or the Fresh Network in the UK.

Chapter 10

The bad

Ah, where to start? You already know my opinion of inorganic synthetic supplements that are chemically manufactured and only guess at the quantities of nutrients that we might require. All of these will fit into the 'bad' category. Additionally some pharmaceutical preparations can be considered under this heading.

Biphosphonates

A group of drugs widely prescribed for osteoporosis is the biphosphonates. These medications owe their mechanism of action to their inhibition of osteoclasts, cells which break down old worn-out bone and eliminate it. This action, on the face of it, might appear to be beneficial, since it will in theory increase bone strength by preventing bone from being broken down. However, as it transpires, it isn't quite that simple. A counter-argument prevails that the osteoclasts know what they are doing, and they are breaking down that old, worn-out bone for a good reason. By taking biphosphonates, and keeping worn-out bone as part of skeletal structure, we are potentially doing our bone health a rather large disservice. In fact, a listed side effect of biphosphonates is a reduction in bone formation by over 70 per cent; surely the opposite of what we are trying to achieve. There are other rather nasty potential side effects, including, but not restricted to:

Hypocalcaemia (reduction in calcium levels)
Increased parathyroid hormone levels
Skin rash
Atrial fibrillation (a heart problem, for which further drugs, and anticoagulants, will be prescribed)
Bone pain

Fractures of the femur (thigh bone)
Gut irritation
Oesophageal ulceration and oesophageal cancer
Osteomalacia
Hyperphosphataemia (excessive phosphorus levels)
Jaw osteonecrosis (death of the jaw bone).

Reading through this list, it really does make one wonder why this category of medication is one of the mainstays of treatment for osteoporosis. If used for longer than five years, it actually increases the risk of fractures, particularly fractures of the femur. At the 2014 conference of the American Society for Bone and Mineral Research, the adverse effects of biphosphonates were discussed in detail, and one lecture was specifically aimed at the pros and cons of these drugs, and how the 'risk to reward' ratio for each patient should be carefully considered prior to prescribing them. Newer drugs, discussed below, might mean that eventually biphosphonates are phased out as a treatment for osteoporosis.

As a result of some of the side effects of biphosphonates, other prescription medications might be considered necessary to counteract them, and this could be particularly detrimental to bone building in the future. A common one relates to atrial fibrillation, a condition in which the muscles in the smaller and, thankfully, less important heart chambers stop contracting properly. Atrial fibrillation leads to an increased risk of blood clots, and people with this disease are not only put onto heart medication, but also might be prescribed the anticoagulant warfarin, which is fundamentally a type of rat poison. As a result of taking warfarin, vitamin K is blocked, and patients are told not to eat any foods containing high levels of vitamin K, since this might disturb the blood levels and action of warfarin. Unfortunately this advice involves avoiding foods such as green leaves, and many others that are beneficial for bone health (see chapter 9). Since we already know how important vitamin K is for bone health, and that the foods containing good levels of vitamin K also contain calcium, magnesium, folic acid and many other bone-healthy minerals, can you appreciate how this might lead to a downward spiral, particularly detrimental to building bone strength in the long term?

Steroid drugs

Corticosteroids have already been mentioned with reference to their detrimental effect on bone density. They reduce calcium absorption and therefore if used in the long term for whatever medical reason (e.g. asthma, allergies, some types of arthritis), they increase our likelihood of osteoporosis. They definitely deserve to be in the 'bad' category.

Fluoride

Fluoride is still being seen as a cure for all dental problems. There is a big debate going on in my home city right now as to whether fluoride should be added to our drinking water to prevent dental caries. There was, in the 1980s, some interest in fluoride regarding whether it might be useful as a treatment for osteoporosis. Fluoride, claimed the proponents, increased the apparent bone density when viewed on X-rays and DEXA scans. However, the 'denser' bone was actually of very poor quality, most probably due to fluoride's adverse effects on the integrity of collagen, one of the structural proteins in bone which was discussed in chapter 2. Fluoride was later found to increase the risk of hip fractures, so its use fell out of favour about 25 years ago. This is a further example of how DEXA scans are only part of the picture regarding bone quality, strength and resistance to fractures.

Fluoride also has other sinister side effects. It plays a role in sleep disorders by accumulating in the pineal gland in the brain and reducing the levels of melatonin, a hormone necessary for good-quality sleep. As you'll read in chapter 11, it's essential to get plenty of rest to boost one of your bone-building hormones. Empirical research from top universities has also indicated that fluoride alters the immune response by inhibiting antibody formation, and the Environmental Protection Agency has linked fluoride consumption to cancer. Fluoride is also reported to cause degeneration of nerves, kidney disease in animals and birth defects, as a result of alteration of brain function and hormones in the foetus.

Fluoride is an incredibly toxic by-product of the agricultural fertiliser industry and one of the problems we have with it is that it cannot be stored, because it is so potent it eats through any storage containers it is placed in, even those made from reinforced concrete. So, an excellent solution is to allow governments to trickle it into the drinking water supply, informing you that it reduces dental caries in children and that it may make your bones stronger. It absolutely does not. It is a poison that was used during the holocaust to render prisoners sterile. It has no place in the human system, especially not in toothpaste, and recent studies have shown that it has no effect on the incidence of dental caries. We must put up vehement opposition to anyone wanting to contaminate our water supply with this dangerous chemical. If you have further concerns regarding fluoride, please look up the Fluoride Action Network for more information.

Diuretics

Water retention, an accumulation of tissue fluid which can cause swelling and bloating of the abdomen, ankles and hands, is treated medically in some people by using diuretics, and these drugs cause problems with bone density. All diuretics, by acting on the part of the kidney structure responsible for resorption of water, have the unfortunate effect of increasing the rate of urinary calcium loss, even those considered to be 'calcium-sparing'. The age group normally treated with diuretic drugs tends to be the elderly, since diuretics are used to treat congestive heart disease and hypertension (high blood pressure). As always, the underlying causes should be addressed. Hypertension is easy to reverse through a plant-based diet, avoidance of alcohol and by using appropriate wholefood supplementation.

Salt

Excessive salt consumption is being linked with the increased risk of developing osteoporosis. Studies conducted prior to the new millennium describe any correlation as 'debatable', but more recently published literature indicates salt as a common link to high blood pressure and osteoporosis, due to its effect on increasing calcium loss via the urine. This urinary calcium loss induces a negative calcium balance that may predispose hypertensive subjects to developing greater bone loss over time.[2]

The downright ugly

Is there anything that really deserves to be put in this category? In my opinion, absolutely yes! There is one very widely used supplement available that to my mind should carry a skull and crossbones on its label. It is, admittedly, never touted as a supplement that will build strong bones, but it is widely used, and even recommended, for the treatment of arthritis. It is commonly available in practically every health food store, throughout Europe and North America. Intelligent people still choose to consume it daily. It is...

Cod liver oil

How can this be? Granny used it all the time didn't she? Well, maybe she did, and I won't lie to you, it is a good food source of vitamin D. But, unlike *Sun D* mentioned above, it comes with a whole stack of detrimental properties associated with it. Firstly, any sea-dwelling creature near the top of the food chain is going to concentrate toxins in its system, as a result of the widespread pollution that we have subjected our oceans to. This is why many health experts are now in agreement that we should be eating low on the food chain. Cod is a large fish that is fairly high on the food chain, and there are two major contaminants likely to be present in cod that we absolutely do not want in our bodies. The first of these is mercury. Mercury is one of the top three most toxic elements on the planet. It damages the central nervous system, endocrine system and kidneys. Prolonged ingestion over a period of time can lead to brain damage and death.

The second toxin which specifically accumulates in the liver of these fish is organophosphate. Organophosphates are a common pollutant from the agrochemical industry, and run-off has long been known to be polluting our rivers, and therefore ultimately the sea. Again, these herbicides concentrate higher up the food chain. Organophosphates damage our nervous system by interfering with acetyl cholinesterase at the synaptic junction of our nerves; in other words, preventing communication of 'messages' being transported along the nerves. Clearly, we do not want the transmission of our nerve impulses interfered with.

These toxins are all very well, you might say, but what about using 'pure, uncontaminated' cod liver oil? Realistically, as a result of oceanic pollution, there is no such thing. But my disapproval of the use of cod liver oil goes deeper, particularly in relation to osteoporosis. It is being shown to be a factor in the deterioration of our bone strength. Yes, cod liver oil contributes to osteoporosis, and therefore has no place in the human diet. Many studies have linked the very high incidence of osteoporosis in Scandinavia to the widespread use of cod liver oil. The reason? This toxic supplement contains very high levels of vitamin A.

Vitamin A weakens our bones as a result of its inhibitory effect on osteoblasts, the cells that form new bone. It has also, at high dose rates, been indicated to interfere with vitamin D, which we know is beneficial for bone health, and with low levels adversely affecting other bodily systems. Even if you have not been diagnosed with osteoporosis, do yourself a big favour and *never* take cod liver oil.

Antacids

TV advertising has a lot to answer for, wouldn't you say? The 'cure' for inappropriate eating is, apparently, not to make better food choices, but to take antacids to relieve ourselves of the symptoms of eating inappropriate non-foods that our body is desperately asking us not to do, by giving us discomfort when we do it. Antacids, in relation to osteoporosis, are potentially a disaster.

Firstly, many of the nutrients we need to absorb for building our bone strength are best absorbed in the presence of strong gastric hydrochloric acid (HCl), notably calcium, copper and folic acid. Many of us, particularly when we reach the age that is generally associated with osteoporosis, have low levels of hydrochloric acid in our stomachs. There are many ways in which this can be addressed, which I recommend that you look into. A full discussion is slightly outside the scope of this publication, but drinking water with lemon juice and a pinch of cayenne pepper each morning is one recommended method. You'll find more information about testing for low gastric HCl levels in my previous book, *The Whole Body Solution*. Increasing gastric HCl will improve your digestion and assimilation of many important nutrients, not just those responsible for bone health.

Several brands of antacid also contain another very damaging element, and that is aluminium. Aluminium, in addition to being linked to Alzheimer's and dementia, is connected with osteoporosis. Aluminium accumulates in bone, inhibiting new bone formation and increasing bone resorption. It also promotes urinary calcium loss, as well as binding phosphorus in the digestive tract (phosphorus is an essential component of bone crystals). Animal studies have shown that consumption of aluminium compounds leads to osteoporosis. Aluminium, for its part, is also present in canned carbonated drinks (which have already been discussed in chapter 4), in underarm deodorants, and in cooking pots – another reason to eat your food uncooked. It is additionally present in food additives, another reason to avoid all processed food.

Antacid manufacturers, however, would have you believe that their products are good for you because they contain calcium. Indeed they do, but it is not a form of calcium that you can benefit from, and they contribute to calcium loss, so nothing could be further from the truth. Eliminate the perceived need for antacids and improve your digestion by eating a mostly raw, plant-based alkalising diet, following the principles of good food combining to avoid digestive stress. Seek out a good raw food coach in your area to guide you in this. It would also be beneficial to use digestive enzymes with each meal if you suffer from poor digestion and associated heartburn.

Alcohol

Make no mistake: alcohol is a drug, and a rather dangerous one at that. In addition to destroying liver and brain cells via its breakdown pathway which produces acetaldehyde (chemically similar to formaldehyde), it has been demonstrated to be exceptionally damaging to bone health. According to the National Institute on Alcohol Abuse and Alcoholism (NIAAA), alcohol interferes with calcium and bone metabolism in several ways. Acute alcohol consumption can lead to a transient parathyroid hormone deficiency and increased urinary calcium excretion, resulting in a loss of calcium from the body. Chronic heavy drinking disturbs vitamin D metabolism, with the negative effects that vitamin D deficiency can produce, as discussed in the previous chapter. Regular consumption of alcohol also interferes with vitamin C absorption.

Further data from the NIAAA reports that studies in alcoholics show that alcohol is directly toxic to bone-forming cells and inhibits their activity. In addition, chronic heavy drinking can adversely affect bone metabolism indirectly, for example by contributing to nutritional deficiencies of calcium or vitamin D. Liver disease and altered levels of reproductive hormones, both of which can be caused by alcohol, also affect bone metabolism. In alcoholics, the risk of osteoporosis is substantially increased.[3]

Studies with abstinent alcoholics have found that alcohol-induced changes in bone metabolism, including toxic effects on bone-forming cells, are at least partially reversible after cessation of drinking, so it appears that it's never too late to adjust your lifestyle habits to protect the integrity of your bone health.

Antidepressants

The most commonly prescribed antidepressants are those with the classification of SSRIs (selective serotonin reuptake inhibitors), such as Prozac, Zoloft and Paxil. They inhibit the protein that transports the hormone and neurotransmitter serotonin; this protein has also been found in bone. Preliminary studies indicate that SSRI antidepressants may interfere with both osteoblasts and osteoclasts, and may also have a directly damaging effect on bone. This is supported by in vitro testing. Serotonin in the gut has been found to have an inhibitory action on bone formation, so any drug which makes serotonin last longer in the body, such as SSRIs, could have detrimental effects on overall bone strength.

There is massive pressure from the pharmaceutical companies to get people onto antidepressants, it would appear. I am not a great one for responding to advertising questionnaires on the internet, but I couldn't resist this one. 'Are you at risk of depression?' it asked. 'Take our 5 minute test and find out.' So I did the questionnaire. I answered 'no' to all 10 questions; I am not in the slightest at risk of depression in my opinion. When my 'professional analysis' of my answers came back, I was little short of horrified. 'You might be at risk of depression. Ask your doctor if "Drug X" might be right for you.' What total nonsense; I had answered no to every single question – I am one of the least 'at risk of depression' people I can think of. Fortunately, I have the knowledge and scientific training not to be taken in by such rubbish. Please be very careful. Advertising can be extremely insidious and lead you to believe that you may have a problem when none exists. Just because vast numbers of women go through life on SSRIs it does not mean that this is a normal state of affairs. It is very far from healthy. And since SSRIs are known to increase the risk of suicide, how can they be considered to cure a problem?

SSRIs are controversial at best in relation to treatment of depression. Sadly, women who are depressed are at greater risk from osteoporosis in the first instance, according to recent studies, so prescribing SSRIs to them is likely to make matters worse. No one would argue that depression is a potentially serious problem, but surely a better way would be to boost mood, and bone density, with regular exercise? In fact, recent studies have shown that exercising for just 20 minutes a day is a more effective treatment for mild to moderate depression than *any* currently available prescription antidepressant. Supplementation is also potentially beneficial, although more research needs to be conducted in this area. Blue-green algae contain compounds which have been shown to elevate mood, notably phenylethylamine (PEA). For more help regarding the serious issue of depression, I recommend reading *Depression Free for Life* by Dr Gabriel Cousens.

Chapter 10

Other drugs used to treat osteoporosis

You will probably have concluded by now that I am not a great fan of pharmaceutical intervention for osteoporosis, when so many natural methods have been proven to be effective. Some anti-osteoporotic drugs might play a small part in increasing bone density, but as we now know from chapter 2, this is not necessarily an indication of reduced fracture risk, although some drugs are claimed to reduce fracture risk by 50 per cent. Some drugs can be useful for those in imminent danger of bone fractures, whilst waiting for the benefits of lifestyle and dietary changes and supplementation regimes to take effect, but I do not see them as a long-term solution. Likewise, anti-osteoporotic drugs will definitely not create bone *health,* and also come with a host of potential side effects which cause problems elsewhere in the body, as seen above for the biphosphonates. There is a big difference between these two concepts.

Selective oestrogen receptor modulators (SERMs)

This drug category is not a hormone but has the effect of mimicking the effect of oestrogen in bone tissue, and elsewhere in the body. The most famous drug in this category is tamoxifen, which is used in the treatment of breast cancer. As we will discuss in chapter 11, the hormone most likely to be beneficial to bone building is not oestrogen but progesterone, making me question why this category of drug is suggested for osteoporosis treatment. Its side effects include elevation in certain types of blood fats, thereby possibly increasing cardiovascular risk; it also increases the risk of blood clots and cancer of the uterus.

Parathyroid hormone treatment

Parathyroid hormone (PTH) is responsible for the regulation of blood calcium levels and is a recognised drug treatment for osteoporosis. Stated to strengthen bone and reduce fracture risk, it is given as a daily injection and is more expensive than other treatments. According to the National Osteoporosis Society, it is more likely to be used in people who have already sustained a fracture. Side effects include nausea, limb pain, headaches, dizziness, lowering of blood pressure and depression. It cannot be used in people who have liver or kidney problems.

Human monoclonal antibody treatment (RANK-ligand inhibitors)

These are new treatments which are based upon inhibiting sclerostin. Sclerostin is a protein that's produced by the osteocytes (the cells buried in the bone matrix), which inhibits the activity of osteoblasts, the bone-building cells that were described in chapter 2. Sclerostin exists to prevent the bones from becoming too bulky. The theory behind these RANK-ligand inhibitor drugs is that we want to knock out anything that is inhibiting the activity of bone-building cells; by doing so we can better maintain bone mass. Since sclerostin is specific to bone tissue, it has been suggested that drugs which work by inhibiting its action will have fewer side effects. A natural method of inhibiting the action of sclerostin is load-bearing exercise, the importance of which is discussed in chapter 12, and the action of parathyroid hormone when adequately in balance.

In a recent study, romosozumab, a RANK-ligand inhibitor which is currently in stage three clinical trials, was demonstrated to be associated with increased bone mineral density and formation, and decreased bone resorption in post-menopausal women with low bone density.[4] Despite the specificity for sclerostin, there are side effects associated with the use of RANK-ligand inhibitors, which include urinary infection, chest infection, cataract, constipation, skin rashes, eczema, sciatica and limb pain. Despite this, it is still stated to be a 'well-tolerated' drug.

Chapter 10 summary

- Many readily available supplements are ineffective and have no bone health benefits. Only use wholefood derived supplements.
- Many pharmaceutical prescription drugs have adverse effects on bone strength in the long term. These include anti-osteoporosis biphosphonate drugs, steroids, antidepressants and antacids.
- Cod liver oil is toxic and should never be used.
- Alcohol is a poison which has many adverse health effects, including weakening of the bones.
- There are new drug treatments being developed for osteoporosis, but they still have the potential to lead to adverse side effects. Weight-bearing exercise has the same benefit as these drugs, without the side effects.

Chapter 11

Chill out and let go – the fascinating world of hormones and stress

The adrenal hormones

How to reduce stress and give the adrenals a break

Could it be that we are indeed exposed to 50 times the abnormal stress levels that we were even 60 years ago? I have no doubt that life can be stressful. We want it all, we want it now and we seem to be forced into being consummate overachievers. Women have to juggle work, children and relationships. Men still feel they have to be the main provider and we are collectively being drawn into the negative spiral of having to be seen to have more, do more, spend more... Advertising tells our children, and we ourselves, that our lives will not be complete without the latest expensive gadget, which of course costs money that would perhaps be better spent on buying better quality food.

I realise that there will always be different personality types. I, for example, am a self-confessed Type A. No one had to drive me to achieve, I did that myself. This overachievement mentality brings with it inevitable stress – stress that you will miss deadlines, stress that you will not be good enough, stress that you will not receive recognition. In this kind of environment, is it any wonder that our innate 'fear, fight and flight' mechanism is being continually overworked, leading to adrenal exhaustion and depression? It is very easy for me to sit here and say 'Chill out and let go'; you might feel unable to. My late father had a lovely saying which went as follows: 'In 100 years' time none of this will matter.' Of course he was right, since not many of us will still be around in 100 years. So let's address this now.

How stress affects the bones and the whole body

There are two main hormones governing the stress reaction: cortisol and adrenaline. They work together to exert the 'fear, fight and flight' response that was first described in the scientific literature as long ago as 1936. This response gives a temporary increase in energy production, at the expense of processes that are not required for immediate survival. The resulting biochemical and hormonal imbalances should ideally resolve as soon as the danger is over, due to a hormonally driven negative feedback loop. The following is a typical example of how the stress response is supposed to operate as a survival mechanism:

An individual is faced with a stressor.
A complex hormonal cascade ensues, and the adrenals secrete cortisol.
Cortisol prepares the body for a fight-or-flight response by flooding it with glucose, supplying an immediate energy source to large muscles.
Cortisol inhibits insulin production in an attempt to prevent glucose from being stored, favouring its immediate use.
Cortisol narrows the arteries whilst adrenaline increases heart rate, increasing the blood pressure and delivering more oxygen-rich blood to the tissues.
The individual addresses and resolves the situation.
Hormone levels return to normal.

Unfortunately, with our over-stressed, fast-paced lifestyle, our bodies are pumping out cortisol almost constantly, which wreaks havoc on our health. In times of high stress the body will break down amino acids to form glucose through the process of gluconeogenesis (a physiological process via which proteins and amino acids are utilised, instead of glucose), to produce energy. Cortisol is the major stress hormone that promotes this process. Collagen, being a structural tissue made from protein, is one of the target areas for spare amino acids; the muscles are another. Chronically elevated stress levels increase collagen breakdown. Since collagen is the matrix upon which our bones are built, anything that is likely to break it down will have potentially serious consequences for the strength and integrity of the bones.

Cortisol primarily acts on the outer layer of the bone, known as the periosteum. Research has shown that elevated cortisol levels interfere with the formation of osteoblasts and cell proliferation.[1] This dramatically decreases bone building and lowers bone density. Without adequate rest and repair, bone mineralisation and collagen formation will be reduced for the duration of the elevated stress. Remember also from chapter 9 that the absorption of vitamin D is adversely affected by high cortisol levels. This gives a double whammy in favour of bone loss.

Stress, as I have mentioned, can rot your bones faster than a can of fizzy drink. Stress and the negative emotions that accompany it have been shown to have a chemical structure in our bodies. And guess what? That chemical structure is acidic! With all the emphasis I placed on ensuring appropriate intake of alkaline minerals in earlier chapters, and the fact that increased acidity causes increased urinary calcium excretion (see chapter 4), is it any wonder that for prevention and reversal of osteoporosis we absolutely *have* to take stress reduction seriously?

The power of exercise

My favourite way of combating the stress that often accompanies a bad day at work is to get out and go for a run, or go to a karate class. Both are also excellent ways of not only de-stressing the body but also positively stressing the bones to increase bone strength. Exercise is a surefire way to de-fuse. It boosts the level of endorphins in the brain, morphine-like 'happy hormones' which are often depleted by our daily lives. Relaxation classes and guided meditation are well worth doing, as is a meditation based on love and compassion. Thoughts of love and compassion stimulate the production of a hormone called oxytocin, whose effects in the body work in the opposite way to those of cortisol. Oxytocin lowers the blood pressure and relaxes the walls of the arteries.

Breathe deeply

Breathwork will reduce stress levels, as will walking in nature. Even better, why not walk in nature with man's best friend? This could be beneficial not just because brisk walking is good for bone density, but pet ownership has also been shown to reduce blood pressure in susceptible individuals.[2] However, before rushing out and buying or adopting a pet animal please make sure that you have the means, financial and otherwise, to look after it properly. In my 30-year-long role as a veterinarian I have had to euthanise many animals because their owners could not, or chose not to, pay for the care they needed.

Whatever you do to reduce stress, ensure that you enjoy it and that it will suit your personality type. If you have to force yourself to go to a meditation class you might be fidgeting all the way through and not receive any benefit, and possibly even make yourself more stressed as a result. I for one confess to not being very good at sitting still in meditation and concentrating on my breathing. That is why running sprint intervals and doing karate serves me well for chilling out and letting go. In fact, over the years, running has become my way of meditating. We're all different, so work out what works best for you. Yoga, for example, is great for relaxation if you choose one of the gentler styles. Choose a more dynamic style for better bone-building results. Do not, whatever you do, let stress or resentment build up inside you, because it will insidiously eat away at your bones.

Good old magnesium

In addition to its beneficial effect on bone health (see chapter 8), magnesium is a mineral that we hear a lot about in relation to stress. The good news about a plant-based diet high in greens, particularly one that emphasises the use of green juices and wheatgrass juice every day, is that it will contain decent levels of magnesium.

The sex hormones

Following on from mentioning the hormones cortisol, adrenaline and endorphins, it's now time to talk about the sex hormones. Bone loss in women accelerates faster after the menopause, so let's have a closer look at the hormones that are responsible for bone health, and how we can optimise their effects.

There are a total of six sex hormones that play a part in bone strength, so I continue to be surprised that the main one women still hear about is oestrogen; oestrogen is actually the least important, even to the point of being detrimental (see page 130).

These six hormones are:

Oestriol
Oestradiol
Oestrone
Progesterone
DHEA
Testosterone

At menopause, women often agonise over the decision as to whether to take hormone replacement therapy (HRT). They hear that it could prevent the undesirable effects of menopause, such as hot flushes, night sweats and accompanying unpleasantness, but have not been made aware of the potential ill-effects of synthetic hormones, such as increasing their risks of breast cancer and stroke. Synthetic hormones seem to be prescribed so commonly it remains a mystery to me as to why the patient's baseline hormone levels never seem to be tested first, to assess which ones are needed, whether they are needed, and if so, in what ratios. Before you begin dabbling in hormone treatments, even if they are the 'safe' bioidentical type, make sure that you get a blood test. Hormones are potent chemicals that are not to be taken lightly or indiscriminately; it is essential that you are tested for the levels of all of these hormones and that the ratios of each are considered. Just as with minerals, overdoing it with one hormone can cause very serious consequences with others.

Let's have a look at the hormones now and the effects they have on bone strength.

The oestrogens

Oestriol, oestradiol and oestrone are all oestrogens, hormones that are produced by the ovaries. Until menopause, they are considered to have a protective effect on bone density and also reduce the incidence of cardiovascular disease. Falling oestrogen levels after the menopause are quoted as one of the reasons that women have a greater incidence of cardiovascular disease once the menopause has occurred.[3]

It has been observed that in the three to four years after menopause, bone loss takes place more rapidly, at a rate of 3 to 4 per cent per year, then it slows down again to a loss rate of 1 to 1.5 per cent per year. As a result, it has been almost universally accepted that this accelerated rate of bone loss must be as a result of the decline of oestrogens. However, it is somewhat more complicated than that, and some researchers now are suggesting that the increased bone loss is as a result of a 'correction' in an oestrogen level that was artificially high in the first place. According to Dr George Yu, senior physician at Aegis Medical and Research Associates (Annapolis, Maryland), it is the more rapid drop in progesterone at this time that is likely to be responsible for this loss in bone mass, rather than the oestrogen, and brings about the concept of oestrogen dominance (see below). Indeed, one of the consistent findings with those consuming a plant-based diet, compared with those whose diets contain high levels of animal products, is that the plant-eaters have lower levels of oestrogen (as highlighted by T. Colin Campbell, author of *The China Study*).

Oestrogen dominance

The hormonal systems are in delicate balance, and it is very easy for them to be thrown out of their normal equilibrium, particularly in our modern-day world. One of the concepts that we are now well aware of is that of, in women, oestrogen dominance. The rapid fall in progesterone at the time of menopause skews the ratio of progesterone to oestradiol, leaving oestrogen as the more dominant hormone. However, other external factors are also at play, as a result of the recent surge in levels of environmental oestrogens or xenoestrogens – artificial oestrogens which mimic the natural hormones and compete for their receptor sites. Anyone who regularly consumes commercially produced meat will be exposed to a multitude of artificial hormones, since they are used as growth promoters. Now of course the levels of growth promoters do come under regulation, but realistically we do not know how long their residue is present in the meat and milk of these animals, and just how much they can affect our easily disturbed hormonal equilibrium. You can find more information on xenoestrogens in my previous book, *The Whole Body Solution*.

To conceive or not?

Women are generally more at risk from exposure to artificial hormones as a result of the widespread use of birth control pills. As it stands now, doctors are reminding us that we should not be using birth control pills for any longer than seven years, since the side effects can be far reaching and serious. The contraceptive pill increases the risk of breast and other cancers, heart disease, high blood pressure, vascular disorders including thrombus formation, and infertility once one decides to discontinue their use. Are these risks really worth it? Add to this the fact that the contraceptive pill is usually made from the urine of pregnant horses. Urine drinking as a so-called 'health tool' in some of the more unusual health circles is controversial at best, and that is when the user is imbibing their own urine. Would anyone seriously choose to stand in the firing line of a pregnant mare and deliberately swallow what is voided? But this is how synthetic oestrogens are made, and there is no getting away from the fact that they are not only completely unnatural for humans, but also that the unfortunate horses involved are condemned to a totally miserable life.

Synthetic oestrogens in food

Additionally, synthetic oestrogens are finding their way into the food chain via other means, including, rather alarmingly, via one substance widely touted as a 'health food' – soya (soy) products. I caution against the use of large amounts of soya. Firstly, approximately 98 per cent of it is genetically modified. We are being told by some large corporations that GM food is not only safe, but also the only way we can expect to be able to feed the rapidly expanding global population. I disagree on both counts. Soya products are not healthy. They inhibit thyroid function. They are also potentially responsible for feminisation of men. They are often highly allergenic; food allergies have been proposed to be a contributing factor to the development of osteoporosis. They have, in some studies, been shown to aggravate bone loss and increase breast cancer risk. They may also interfere with the action of progesterone, one of the very important hormones for building of new bone. I would avoid genetically modified soya product use with the same vehemence as dairy products. The health benefits associated with soya can only be attributed to using fermented soya products in condiment quantities, not the unfermented genetically modified products.

Plastics in food and clothes

Plastics are oestrogenic. Food wrapped in plastic will have absorbed some of the oestrogenic potential of the plastic wrapping. Bottled water is being linked with some potentially devastating health consequences, including breast cancer. This is because most plastic bottles leach xenoestrogens into the water they contain, and we subsequently consume it. Even clothes made from plastics (synthetic fibres derived from the petrochemical industry) could allow plastic to be absorbed through the skin that these clothes are in contact with.

Oestrogen – good or bad?

As a result of all this cumulative exposure to xenoestrogens, some demographic studies have indicated that 2 per cent fewer male babies are being born than females. This is an alarming trend. But ultimately, what does all this have to do with osteoporosis? The answer is relatively straightforward: oestrogen dominance. This is such a common state for the premenopausal woman in the developed world that it is now almost being considered to be normal. The trend of, and clinical signs associated with, oestrogen dominance are clearly discussed in the excellent publication *What Your Doctor May Not Tell You About Menopause* by Dr John Lee.

Dr Lee was a great advocate for the use of natural progesterone, which we will be discussing later in this section. So if oestrogen dominance is such a feature of the Western world, why is it that oestrogen replacement is still being considered an appropriate medical treatment for osteoporosis? Even medical texts are not supporting its use. *Scientific American's Updated Medicine Text* (1991), for example, states that 'Oestrogens decrease bone resorption' but 'associated with the decrease in bone resorption is a decrease in bone formation. Therefore, oestrogens should not be expected to increase bone mass.'[4]

This statement was made over 20 years ago, but are we getting the message? If we are, this is only happening very slowly. The pharmaceutical industry still appears to be telling the medical profession to use synthetic oestrogen. And all the time that is happening, we are not doing ourselves any favours. I personally recommend that no one ever takes synthetic hormones. Likewise, I would say never take bioidentical hormones without first having a comprehensive blood hormonal assay performed. We don't know what potentially detrimental effects we may have on our finely tuned hormonal systems by adding in something where it is not needed.

Oestriol

Oestriol has been labelled as 'the oestrogen with no adverse effects' and has been used with some success as a postmenopausal hormone replacement. It does not appear to elevate the risks of cancer in the same way as oestradiol and oestrone, the other two oestrogens. However, it is still only part of the hormone picture, and supplementing, even with a 'harmless' oestrogen when we may already be in a state of oestrogen dominance, seems to have little, if any, validity.

Chapter 11

Marvellous progesterone?

Progesterone is a hormone which is also produced by the ovaries, and can possibly be considered to be the missing link in our hormonal jigsaw with regard to bone density. Osteoblasts, our bone-building cells, possess progesterone receptors, so this fact alone should alert us to the potential role of progesterone in laying down new bone and increasing bone density. Progesterone has also been shown to interfere with the negative effects that corticosteroids have on osteoblasts. During the course of his clinical practice, Dr John Lee treated thousands of women with natural progesterone and noted improvements in their bone density as shown on DEXA scans. In one published study he treated 100 postmenopausal women, who had already had osteoporotic fractures, with natural progesterone. The average increase in bone density was 10 per cent in the first year, with some patients having an increase in bone density of up to 20 per cent. We now know (see chapter 2) that DEXA scans are not necessarily the best way to assess fracture risk, but nonetheless these findings are remarkable, and have never been reproduced with oestrogen treatment or any antiosteoporotic drug. No adverse side effects were demonstrated and the progesterone was well tolerated.

It is still interesting to note, however, that replacing progesterone with natural progesterone cream (it is not well absorbed orally so is used topically onto the skin) is not recognised by the medical profession as a valid osteoporosis treatment, and several researchers have not been able to reproduce the results that John Lee found with his patients. However, when I looked into these studies myself, I found that one of the test groups had more smokers in it, so perhaps this just shows that even the use of bone-building natural progesterone is not fully able to counteract the negative effects of smoking on bone mineralisation.

The importance of progesterone in maintenance of strong

bones is, in my opinion, not in doubt, demonstrated rather nicely by the fact that young female marathon runners can become osteoporotic.[5] Exercise is of course vital for bone strength, but one of the difficulties associated with endurance sport is that particularly the female athletes can end up with very low bodyweight. If a woman drops below 46 kg in weight, she will automatically stop menstruating. This sends progesterone levels plummeting and I have heard of 29-year-old distance runners having osteoporosis, purely because of their lack of hormones. The interesting aspect of studies on marathon runners is that their bone density reduction seems to have little correlation with their oestrogen levels, only that of their progesterone levels, which show a very close correlation. If falling progesterone levels have such a dramatic influence on bone density, leading to osteoporosis in younger women, perhaps we should be focusing more on progesterone levels than oestrogen levels, regardless of age.

Synthetic progesterone, or progestogens, as they are known, have been demonstrated to have beneficial effects on osteoporotic men and women. However, these benefits are not as notable as those obtained with natural progesterone, and by slightly altering the chemical structure of progesterone to make progestogens, we make a compound that has undesirable side effects such as sodium retention, depression, weight gain, nausea, skin rashes and blood clots. Bioidentical hormones are always superior to anything synthetic.

We can obtain natural progesterone via food, and the food with the highest level of progesterone is the wild yam. Oral progesterone, however, is not well absorbed, so if you have been shown to have a low level of progesterone, your bioidentical source will be a cream applied to areas of relatively thin skin. Seek the advice of a doctor trained in bioidentical hormone replacement. I would never recommend that you begin indiscriminately 'supplementing' with natural progesterone cream.

DHEA

DHEA (dehydroepiandrosterone) is a hormone produced by the adrenal glands and the ovaries and has been elevated to the dizzy heights of a 'wonder drug' by some authors. Indeed, when it is suggested that it is of value in treating heart disease, high cholesterol, diabetes, obesity, cancer, Alzheimer's, AIDS and chronic fatigue, it might appear that we have in fact discovered the elusive fountain of youth after all. DHEA levels do decline with age, and it has therefore been postulated that DHEA may play a role in osteoporosis prevention. Breakdown products of DHEA bind to oestrogen receptors, and this may inhibit bone resorption. DHEA is a precursor hormone, which means that it can be converted into other hormones, including oestrogen and testosterone. Although DHEA cannot be directly converted into progesterone, it may elevate progesterone levels via a feedback mechanism involving pregnenolone, from which both DHEA and progesterone are derived.

Thus far, most of the studies on DHEA have been conducted on men, whose incidence of osteoporosis is 10 to 12 per cent that of women. In women, some correlation has been found between bone mineral content and DHEA levels, even after correcting for effects of age. A small-scale trial has indicated statistically significant improvements in bone mineral density in both men and women using DHEA for six months,[6] and there were improvements in body composition in comparison with those who took the placebo. However, in the test subjects it was notable that in addition to elevated DHEA levels, the levels of IGF-1 were also increased, which, as we have learned in chapter 3, has potentially negative implications for health.

Another study has shown that DHEA reverses bone loss in women but not in men. It is also interesting to compare average hormone levels in populations known for their longevity, to normal Western populations of the same age. The population of Okinawa, off southern Japan, has the highest numbers of centenarians per capita than anywhere else in the world. These people enjoy robust health and have a low incidence of degenerative disease, even into advanced age. Their incidence of osteoporosis is also very low. The DHEA levels, for the average 70-year-old woman, is 3 ng/ml (3 nanograms per millilitre of blood), compared to American women of the same age who have just 1.1 ng/ml: almost three times higher. In addition to being beneficial for bone health, these DHEA levels may also reflect a much younger physiological age.

Okinawans eating their traditional diet rich in vegetables and low in animal protein fare much better than those islanders who have now been influenced by the American food industry. Obesity levels and cardiac incidents are now skyrocketing in the younger Okinawans as a result of their unfortunate food choices. I wonder how long it will be before the osteoporosis rate also starts to follow this trend?

Before rushing out to buy the latest DHEA supplement, bear in mind that it is androgenic (stimulates male characteristics) and although generally well tolerated, it can cause acne and stimulate the growth of facial hair. As with all hormones, get tested first to see if you need it. Likewise, if you have, or are at risk from, any of the oestrogen-dependent cancers, DHEA could be contraindicated for you. Get expert advice from a hormone specialist prior to taking any DHEA supplement.

Testosterone

Testosterone is a hormone that women tend to associate exclusively with men, so it is always met with a degree of surprise when I tell a female audience that their bodies also contain testosterone. Testosterone is produced in the female ovary and the male testis, and additionally to a lesser extent in the adrenal glands. After menopause, women generally still have adequate testosterone levels in the blood, but some women fail to produce sufficient. Again, looking at the Okinawans, it appears that the men maintain their testosterone levels for much longer than the average American man; 100-year-old Okinawan men have a similar testosterone reading to that of a 70-year-old American.

Some studies have shown that a combined hormone replacement regime of oestrogen and testosterone has significant benefits for bone density, and more benefit than attributable to just the oestrogen component. However, giving testosterone to women who do not need it is fraught with problems, since it causes masculinisation; you probably don't want to grow a beard if you're female. This is yet another reason for ensuring that you have hormonal tests prior to taking any supplementation.

Balancing the hormones

Hormones are in delicate balance and should never be messed with. By adopting a pure, plant-based diet and maximising the consumption of organic, pesticide-free food whilst avoiding anything oestrogenic, most people will be able to rebalance their hormone systems which play such a vital role in bone density. However, there will always be individuals who are unable to balance their levels through diet and lifestyle alone. For these people, once they have the results of a hormonal assay that tests for all six of the hormones outlined above, bioidentical hormone replacement to correct any deficiency may be appropriate. Seek out an experienced practitioner to help you with this, and above all, never take any synthetic hormone, which could wreak havoc in your delicately balanced system.

HGH – the ultimate fountain of youth?

Aside from the sex hormones mentioned above, there is one very important hormone that might just be considered to be the ultimate 'fountain of youth', and that is human growth hormone (HGH). There have been some placebo-controlled, double-blind studies that indicate the potential use of injections of HGH in the reversal of osteoporosis, and the benefits appear to be dose-dependent.[7] Participants in such studies are generally also taking supplemental synthetic hormones and calcium and/or vitamin D supplementation, so it is difficult to know how much benefit is attributable to the HGH alone. The effect of HGH in bone metabolism seems to be slow in onset and the benefits are lost five years after withdrawal of the injections.

HGH is very expensive, so trials are generally limited due to funding issues. However, since HGH is released in natural 'surges' throughout the day in healthy people, there is a growing interest in whether we can stimulate these natural surges and therefore produce more of our own endogenous HGH; the perfect antidote to the ageing process, without medical intervention. We might be interested in doing this, since HGH stimulates tissue growth, increases muscle tone and lean muscle mass, enhances flexibility and shifts the metabolism to fat-burning mode – something that anyone interested in the maintenance of healthy body weight would be keen to know about.

HGH drops over time, and by the time you reach the age of 60, you produce very little of this anti-ageing hormone. Also, by this age, there is often an accumulation of factors that block its release, which further deplete any benefits. HGH surges can be stimulated by balancing blood sugar (high blood glucose and elevated insulin levels block HGH), avoiding a diet high in processed carbohydrates, performing weight-training exercise, getting adequate, restful sleep and considering having a fasting day once a week (please see my e-book *Successful Fasting for Health and Vitality*, available via www.therawfoodscientist.com, for more information on how to safely conduct a fast). Anaerobic training, i.e. short bursts of high intensity exercise with only short rest periods in between, is best for HGH release. One of the reasons why exercise is so beneficial for bone health relates to its effects on HGH secretion. How appropriate, therefore, that the chapter which follows is devoted to the benefits of exercise.

Is your thyroid working against you?

Finally, before we leave the hormonal section, I want to allay fears about thyroid hormone. Hypothyroidism (an underactivity of the thyroid) seems to be reaching almost epidemic proportions and many people who feel tired and sluggish, and find it difficult to shed excess weight, are often silently going about life with less than optimal thyroid function. The thyroid is a gland in the neck which produces two different thyroid hormones. In *The Whole Body Solution*, also published by Hammersmith Health Books, I outline how best to feed the thyroid so that it performs at its best for you.

Hypothyroidism can be a challenge to diagnose, but once a diagnosis is made, many people turn to supplementation with thyroid hormone to boost the metabolism and regain their zest for life. There have been concerns that by doing this, they put themselves at greater risk of osteoporosis, since an overactive thyroid (hyperthyroidism) is a known aggravator of bone loss. However, there is a big difference between having too much thyroid hormone in the system, and 'topping up' the thyroid levels to where they should be in normality. It appears that bone loss only occurs after a certain level of thyroid hormone is reached in the bloodstream, the likes of which are only seen in true hyperthyroidism, not with supplementation to normalise levels in those with low thyroid readings. Indeed, a study published in *The Lancet* medical journal in 1992 indicated that treatment with thyroid hormone does not cause osteoporosis; neither does it increase the risk of fractures.[8]

Chapter 11 summary

- Stress is hugely detrimental to bone health and must be controlled.
- There are six sex hormones involved in bone health, and they are in delicate balance with each other.
- Synthetic hormones should be avoided. Only natural hormone replacement, under the direction of a knowledgeable practitioner and after careful evaluation of blood samples, should be considered.
- Human growth hormone production can be stimulated naturally through beneficial eating habits and appropriate restful sleep.
- Thyroid hormone supplementation does not seem to be associated with bone loss.

Chapter 12

Exercise – the key to it all?

We're almost there! Before we go any further with our prevention and reversal of osteoporosis information, please bear the following in mind: 75 per cent of the benefit derived from an excellent diet is lost if you don't exercise. You can juice your greens all day long and take your bioavailable wholefood supplements, but if you don't exercise you won't get all the benefits of those foods and supplements. Exercise is great for bones, especially if you do it outside in the sun. You will de-stress, improve your mood, eliminate depression, top up your vitamin D levels and boost your immune system... so get out there if you can, even if you live somewhere cloudy.

Lessons from space

Let's just pause for a minute to think about why exercise is essential for bone strength. Exercise causes our muscles and tendons to pull on our bones. This in turn stimulates new bone to be laid down in the area that is being subjected to this pulling force. As I state in my e-book *Successful Fasting for Health and Vitality* (see chapter 11), we start to lose bone density in our spines within just four days of bed rest. Astronauts, when exposed to conditions of microgravity, are at huge risk of developing osteoporosis because they are in effect weightless, with no external positive stressors on their bones. This is the reason why exercise bikes and other pieces of exercise equipment are provided on the International Space Station (ISS), and the astronauts take their use very seriously, particularly the women.

According to NASA, astronauts give us a very good indication of the benefits of exercise in the reduction of bone loss, since six months at the ISS is the equivalent of what might happen over a five-year time period on Earth. NASA has also been pioneering a test for bone loss that looks at different isotopes of calcium in the urine, which seems to be an accurate determinant of early stages of bone loss which could otherwise go undetected.

Fat bones

Weight-bearing exercise of any description stresses the bones (a beneficial stress, not an adverse one), and this is one of the reasons why it was thought that obese people were less likely to develop osteoporosis. However, a 2013 study by Harvard Medical School has indicated that this might not be the case at all, and that excess fat deposition in the bone marrow of obese people is thought to displace osteoblasts (our bone-building cells), or inhibit their activity. Therefore, ideally, the only weight we should carry on our bodies is muscular weight, not excess fat weight.

What type of exercise?

I am often asked what the best form of exercise is, and my reply is usually the same – the one that you will do! However, that's not quite true for osteoporosis, since if swimming is your preferred exercise, it will not be as beneficial for your bones as lifting weights. Although swimming gives a little benefit for the maintenance of spinal bone mass, most studies have shown that this increased density is not statistically significant. When I tell women they have to lift weights, they are often worried that they will end up looking like bodybuilders. Don't panic – you absolutely will not.

Why do bodybuilders look like they do? Well, usually of course they are male, so they have much more testosterone than women do, a hormone which correlates closely to muscle growth and bulk. Secondly, they often have extreme diets, which could not be further removed from the plant foods regime that I recommend for bone building. Thirdly, they usually take some kind of anabolic steroid or creatine. We've heard of anabolics of course, a banned substance for Olympic athletes, but creatine is becoming a substance advertised to athletes for improving strength and explosive speed. Please avoid it. It causes muscles to take on more water, but the manufacturers seem to have conveniently forgotten that the heart is a muscle, and some young athletes using creatine have died of heart failure. A friend of mine swears that its use made him become an insulin-dependent diabetic. I digress. You will not look like a body builder by doing weight training for another reason as well. The weight training body builders do usually involves lifting extremely heavy weights for only three or four repetitions. I suggest starting off with more repetitions and lighter weights. More weight can gradually be added once you get used to it.

Before we get going with specific exercise recommendations for bone strengthening, it is essential that I mention the obvious. If you have been diagnosed with abnormal blood pressure, or you are an unstable diabetic, or have a specific heart condition, or indeed any other medical condition that might be aggravated by certain types of exercise, it is essential that you talk to your doctor first before beginning any exercise programme, to make sure that it is appropriate for you. If you have not exercised for years you won't be able to do some of the exercises mentioned below. Good technique with a few key exercises is more important than trying to lift weights that are too heavy or for too many repetitions initially, or performing several types of exercise badly, which could put the tendons and ligaments under undue stress.

Likewise, some of these exercises involving weights might

be inappropriate for you if you have been diagnosed with very severe osteoporosis. Whilst someone in that situation may well be able to carefully perform some of the rubber-band exercises shown below, they will not, for example, be able to throw around the 16-kg kettlebell that I use, also shown below. If in doubt, ask an expert before you commence this or any other programme.

Exercise recommendations from an expert

Although I personally love exercise and always train very hard in my sessions, I am not a personal trainer. I am therefore very grateful to Alex Burton, my former personal trainer, for his input into this chapter. Alex is one of the fittest people I know in his age group; he has even completed an Ironman triathlon, a particularly gruelling endurance event which one day I'd like to compete in. I'll let Alex take over from here; I have added a few extra pieces of information below his very helpful recommendations.

The basic principle for maintaining good skeletal bone health from an exercise perspective is to incorporate load-bearing aerobic, resistance and functional exercise.[1] *There is good evidence that applying stress on the bone structures promotes the formation of bone structure.*[2,3,4] *This includes the physical load applied to the bones during muscular contractions. In addition the benefits of increased muscle mass and improved function will aid an individual in minimising the negative impacts of diminished bone density.*

The key is to encourage load bearing in any programme, which is why swimming, although having many fitness benefits, is not the best activity for this purpose. This is why many older people would benefit from less time in the pool, with the exception of pool-based classes that also incorporate hand-held floating weights to add resistance to the workout. These would be a great starting point for people who need more bodily support when beginning an exercise regime.

There is no question that to be really effective, the activity or exercise needs to place the skeleton under 'stress', which is why load-bearing exercises/activities are better. Personally I wouldn't recommend swimming in order to preserve/build bone mass, unless other better options were contraindicated. What is often overlooked is that exercises can be regressed/ progressed to accommodate an individual's needs; for example, the squat progression I mention below. This would have the added benefit of improving overall function/mobility in a key joint movement.

Recommendations fall into two categories:

1. Aerobic activity/exercise

This is predominantly continuous activity which raises heart rate and is movement-based. It benefits the cardiovascular and muscular systems, and it has the added benefit of helping to maintain or improve mobility and coordination.

Perform at least three times per week.

30-60 minutes per session.

Select activities that involve all body movements.

Aim to progress by level of intensity, for example distance covered, time taken to cover a set distance and range of movement or effort.

In this category the best exercise or activity is the one you enjoy and will keep doing with a degree of consistency.

E.g. walking, running (outdoors or indoors on a treadmill), circuit type classes (e.g. Body Pump), indoor rowing, cycling, step machine. Sports such as tennis, badminton, and squash are beneficial, and it is well known that the playing arm of a tennis player has a greater bone density than the non-playing arm.

2. Resistance exercises

The same caveat as above applies regarding fitness to participate in weight-training exercises. It is also important to consider experience/knowledge of correct technique. Good advice here would be to seek guidance from an experienced professional if unsure of any exercise.

If you are new to this type of activity I would advise starting with just using your own bodyweight, or resistance machines before progressing to free weights (dumbbells). However, free weights are likely to provide the greatest benefits.

The best resistance exercises will be large muscle groups and multi-joint, for example ankle, knee, hip.

My recommendations, with progressions/regressions:

I would consider these five key exercises that target the essential movement patterns. The emphasis is on the lower body, which will incorporate whole body stability and core function. Upper body exercises include one pushing/pressing movement and one pulling movement.

SQUATS

Examples – Start with squatting to a seat/bench, either lightly touching or fully seated. Progress to bodyweight only (without the seat), then to light weights, then greater range of movement, then to heavier weights.

Fixed machine leg press could also be used.

Ensure that feet are shoulder-width apart and keep the feet flat on floor. Feel weight in the heels. Bend at hips and knees, keeping chest up and facing forwards. Imagine sitting down and back onto a chair, aiming for a right angle at knees. Make sure that the knees stay pointing slightly outwards, in line with the position of your feet. Avoid the knees folding in on movement.

Return to standing by straightening knees/hips, keeping weight in the feet.

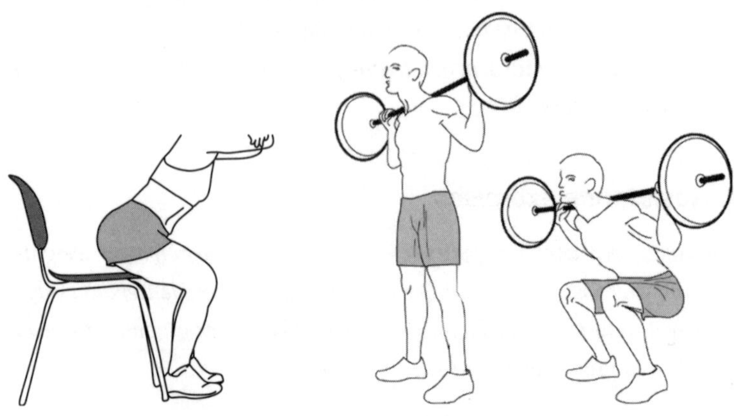

LUNGES

Examples – Alternating leg i.e. from standing, step out forwards, lower rear knee to ground, bend front leg at a right angle, push back with front leg and return to standing. Repeat with the other leg.

Progress to weights, either in each hand or one side only. Progress to walking lunges, i.e. a series of alternate lunges moving forwards instead of returning to standing. Progress to same with weights.

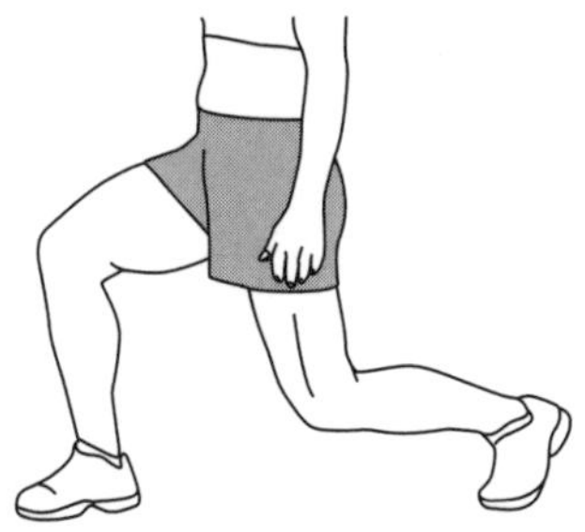

KETTLE BELL SWINGS

Feet hip width apart. Bend at the waist keeping the knees slightly bent. Keep the back as straight as possible, avoiding a curve in the spine.

Hold the kettle bell in both hands with straight arms. Swing by straightening at waist and driving hips forward. Allow weight/arms to swing like a pendulum.

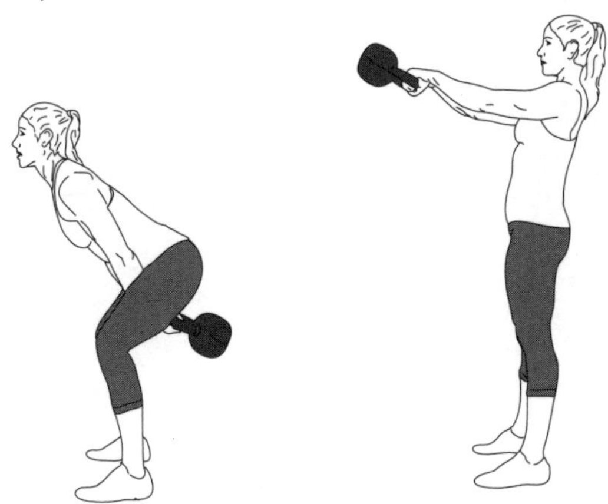

OVERHEAD PRESS

Progress from seated to standing. Using light weights with palms facing forwards (away from you), and elbows pointing out, raise hands from shoulder height to fully extended overhead. Progress by increasing weight to standing, and from there to a weight in one hand.

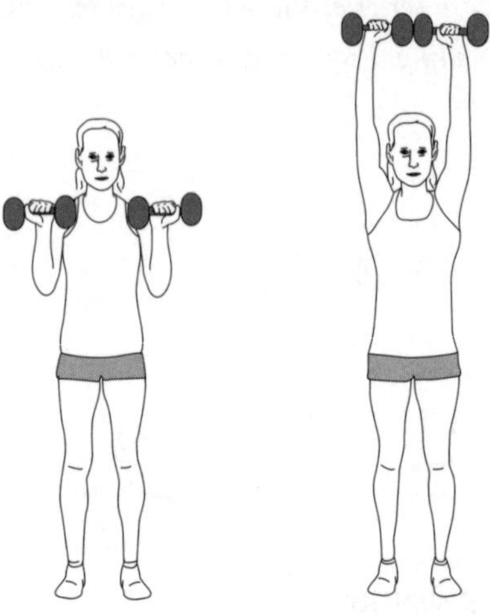

CABLE ROW

Use a fixed cable machine which you'll find at most gyms. Progress from seated to standing or in a semi-squat position. From arm fully extended in front, draw arm back until hand is touching ribs. Keep arm close to body as you draw the cable back.

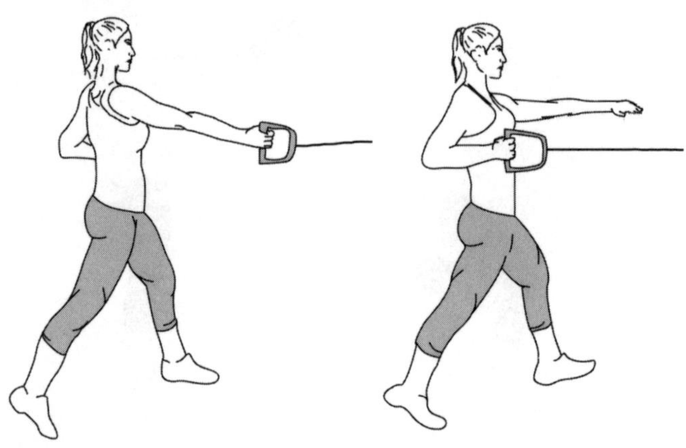

Return slowly controlling weight. Complete one set then repeat with the other arm.

Fixed machine seated row could also be used.

Ideally the above five exercises should be performed three times a week.

Three sets of 10 to 15 repetitions.

Perform at a weight where you feel you could only do three or four more repetitions in each set.

Aim to progress by increasing either the weight, or number of repetitions, or sets over time, for example over a period of three to four weeks. Only change one of these variables at a time.

For all exercises, perform the movement slowly and deliberately. The aim is to control your movement and any additional weight, and this applies to all phases, for example lowering in the squat and returning to standing. A useful tip is to count in your head. A count of either one + one or two + two is a good starting point.

A sample session

Five to 10 minutes of movement to warm up. Aim to raise heart rate and prepare for exercise, using all muscles and joints.

Squats — *Three sets of 12 repetitions (reps)*

Kettle bell swings — *Two sets of 15 reps*

Overhead press — *Three sets of 10 to 12 reps*

Lunges — *Two sets of 12 reps*

Cable row — *Two sets (each arm) of 10 to 12 reps*

10 minutes of warm down.

If you're not a gym member, or even interested in the gym

environment, there are other options you could consider. Outdoor exercise is fun, and the following sequence could be done in a park, as part of a walk or run.

1. *Find a bench or other structure that would allow a squatting exercise onto the bench, either just touching, or to fully seated and back to standing.*
2. *Perform three x 12 to 15 reps, or two x 30 seconds continuous.*
3. *Find a similar structure that allows an alternate step-up onto it. Again a bench might suit depending on height, or a set of steps or tree stump. Watch out for tripping up – look where you're putting your feet!*
4. *Perform alternate set-ups, either three x 12 to 20 reps or for two x 30 seconds.*
5. *If you're able, use either of the previous structures to perform a press-up exercise with feet on the ground and hands on the bench or similar.*

Perform two to three x 10 to 12 reps, or two x 20 seconds continuous.

If you're comfortable with this number look to increase sets, repetitions or time accordingly.

Join the resistance

A friend of mine, Debbie Pentland, is a qualified exercise teacher who specialises in teaching exercise and falls-prevention classes to the elderly in and around the Portsmouth area in southern England. She strongly recommends the use of resistance band exercises, and she has kindly allowed me to include some of her exercises below. The great thing about these bands is that you can do the exercises at home; no gym membership is necessary.

Resistance bands are long rubber bands of varying elasticity, and therefore requiring a greater or lesser force to stretch them; you'll find them in gyms or online, on exercise equipment websites. They are an excellent tool for bone building; some studies have indicated that a comprehensive rubber band workout can increase bone strength by over 10 per cent in just 12 weeks. This improvement was without a change of diet or anything else that we now know to be beneficial for bone health, so just imagine what can be achieved with this type of exercise, combined with all the other factors we have discussed. Falls prevention classes are now being promoted by many local authorities, so contact your local council to find out where your nearest class is. It is well worth joining in; with a good teacher, such as my friend, you'll gain strength and have a really good time in the class, since they're designed to be fun.

Here are some exercises for a resistance band workout. Perform five to six repetitions of all the exercises, three to five times a week, and gradually increase to 10 repetitions. When holding the bands, do not wrap them around your hands – you'll cut off the circulation if you do. Again, always check with your doctor first to ensure that these exercises are appropriate for you.

Hips: Sit on a chair. Hook the band under the foot and lift the knee towards chest. Push your heel towards to floor and hold for a count of five. Repeat with the other leg.

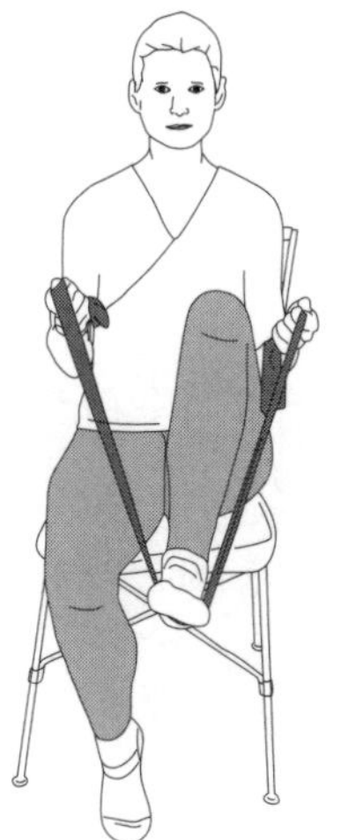

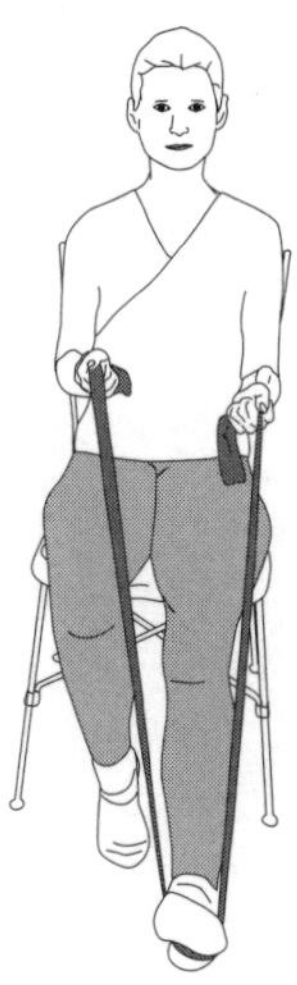

Hips and legs: Sit on a chair with your feet and knees together. Wrap the band around the thighs. Hold the band in place. Move your feet to hip width apart, then push the knees to come into position above the feet, keeping the feet flat on the floor.

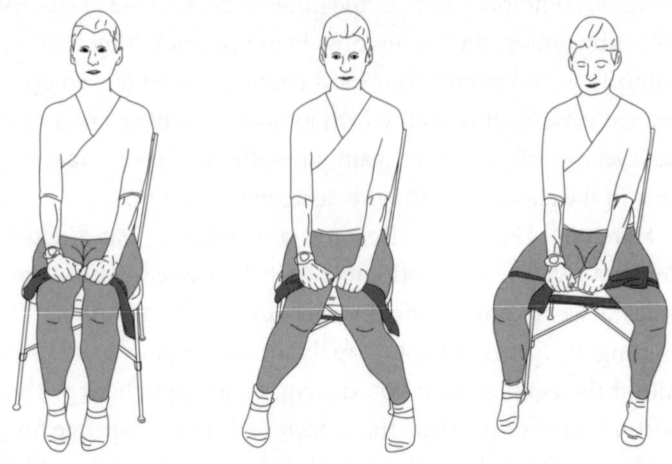

Wrists 1: Roll the band into a cigar shape. Hold it vertically with one hand above the other, elbows out to the sides. Squeeze and twist the band, bringing elbows towards each other.

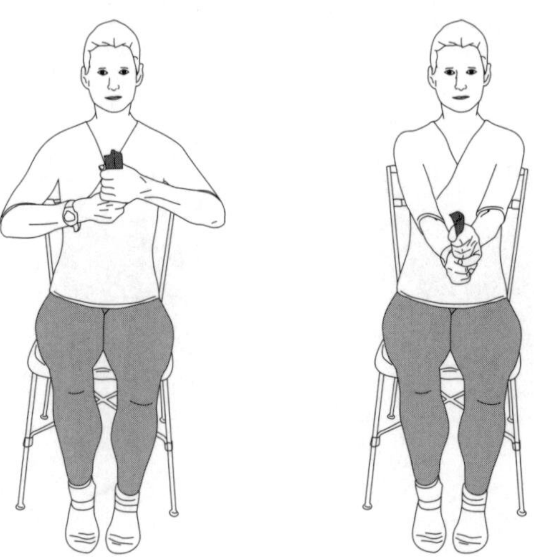

Wrists 2: Hold the rolled-up band horizontally. Try to pull your hands apart.

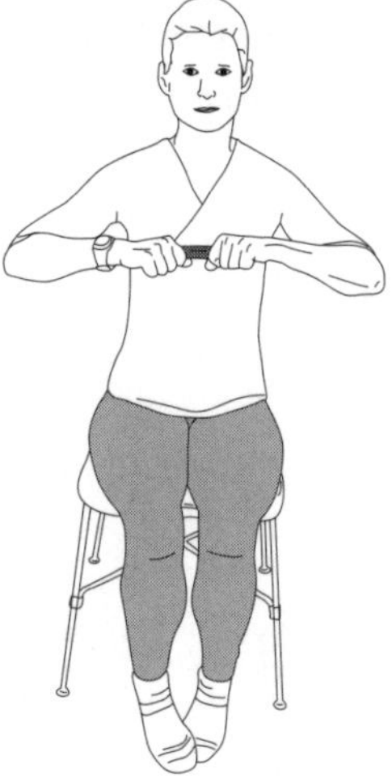

Upper spine: Sit on a chair. Hang the band over your lap and take hold of it with your palms facing upwards. Keeping your elbows touching the sides of your body, pull your hands outwards, holding for a count of five.

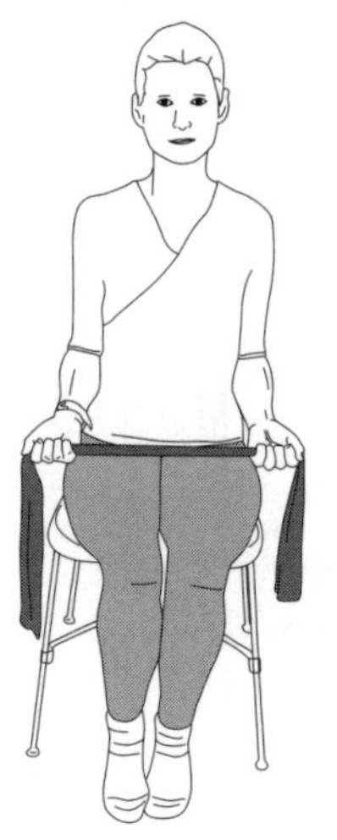

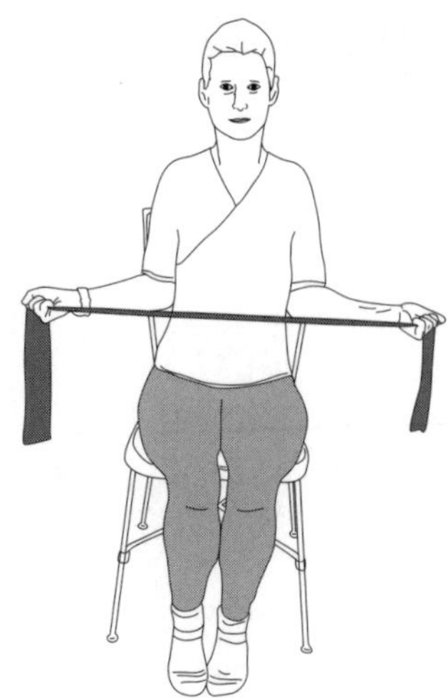

Lower spine: Sit on a chair. Hook the band under both feet. Pull your hands up to rest on the knees. Straighten up the back and relax the shoulders. Tuck the pelvis in and hold for a count of five before releasing. This exercise should give you the feeling of being pushed into a chair.

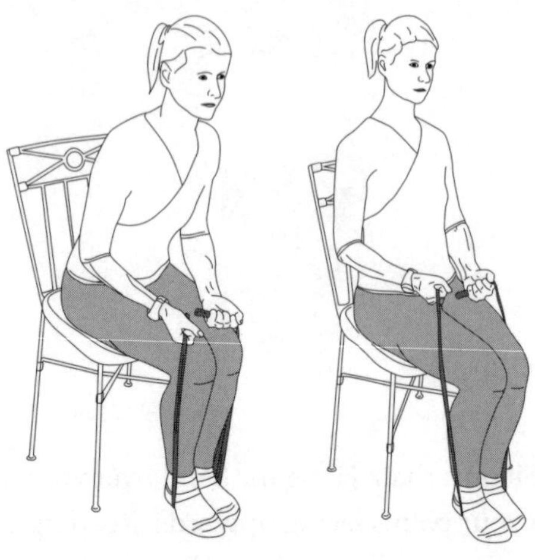

Biceps: Sit on the band and take one end in each hand. Keeping the elbows tucked into the sides of the body, pull the fists up towards the shoulders and release.

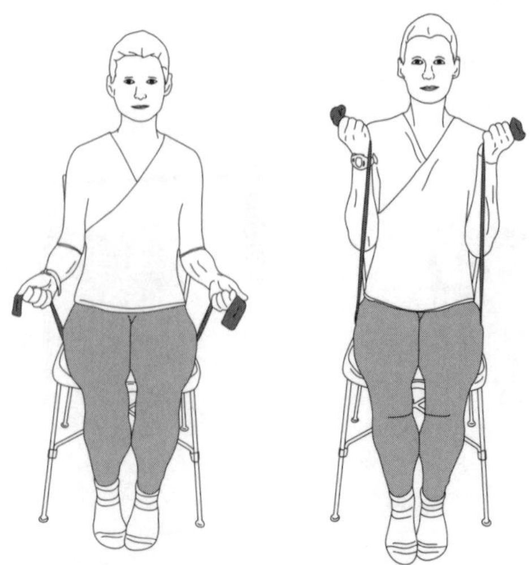

Chest: Sit on a chair. Place the band behind your back and under the arms. Push both arms forwards and cross the arms in front of the chest whilst they are pushed out straight.

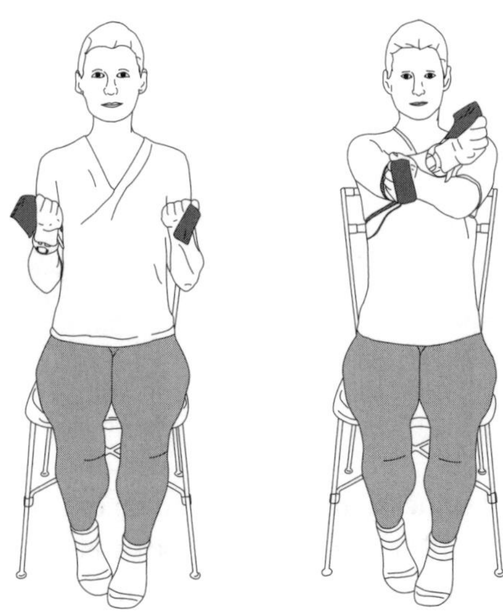

Arms and abdomen: Sit on the floor with your knees bent. Hook the band under both feet and extend your legs. Pull both arms towards and behind you as if rowing. Try not to lean back; sit up tall.

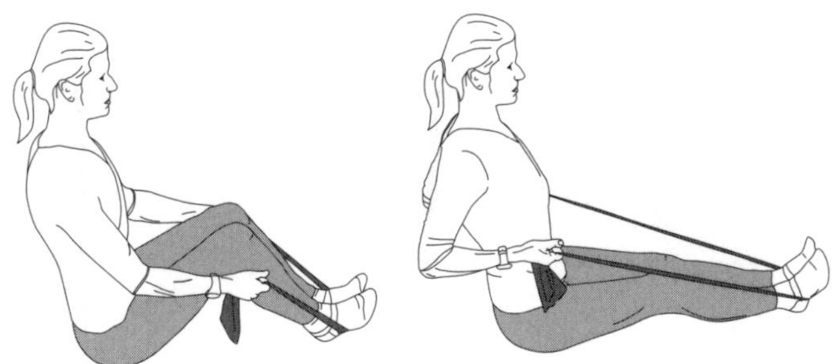

Shoulders and arms: Sit on the band, and take one end in each hand. Lean forward. Lift the arms up and out to the side; release.

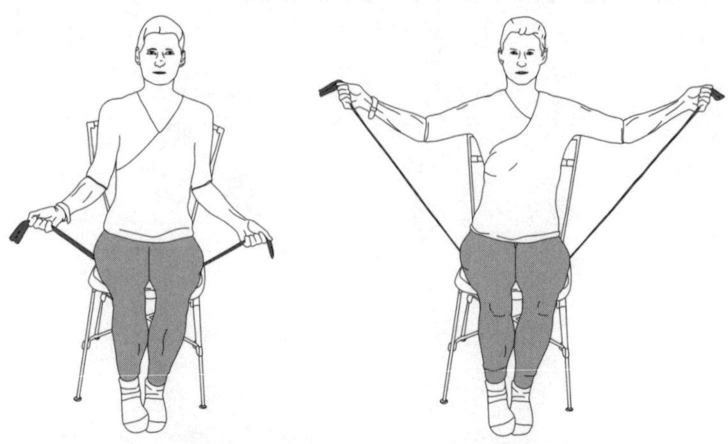

Legs, arms and spine (standing) 1: Stand on one end of the band, with feet hip width apart. Hold the other end in both hands. Bend the knees and then pull the band up to your chin, then nose, then up as high as you can manage. Remember to bend the knees between each pull.

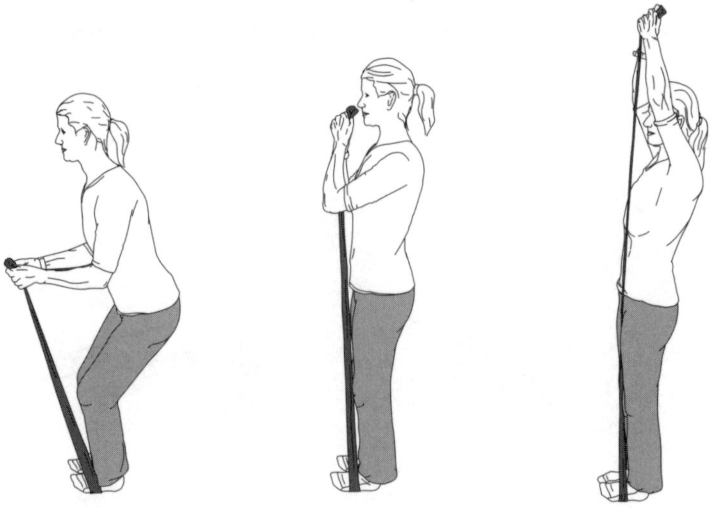

Legs, arms and spine (standing) 2: Start in the same position as above. Hold the band in both hands. Pull up 10 times in 10 different directions. Remember to bend the knees between each pull up.

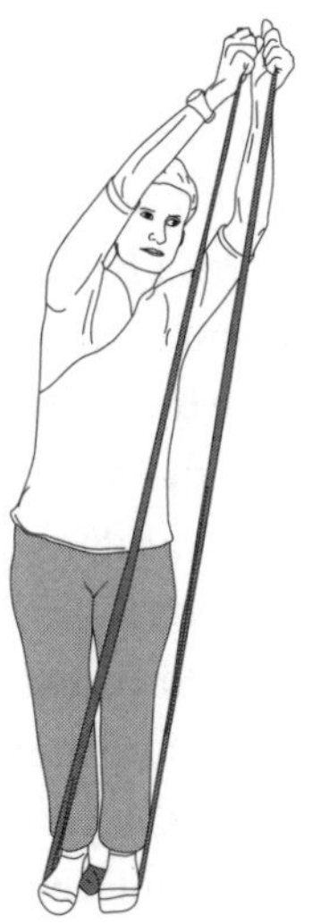

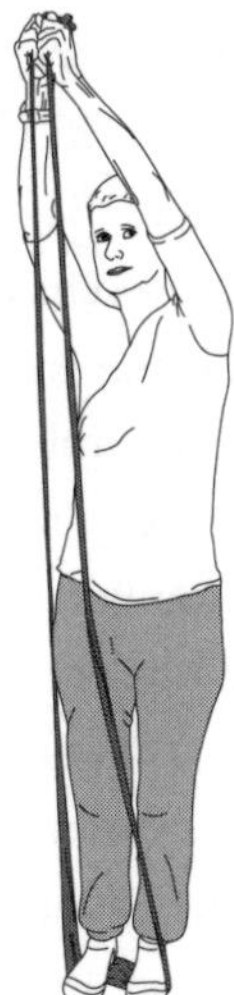

Feel the force

Strength training with weights is absolutely essential to boost growth of new bone. It also has a secondary benefit for those with osteoporosis, whether or not they have already sustained a fracture. It helps to improve balance and coordination, thus making falls less likely, and therefore, in turn, a bone is less likely to fracture if falls are prevented.

Finally on the subject of weight training, it creates a more attractive body as we age. I personally find muscle definition sexy on both men and women. How many times do we see 'bingo wings' on older ladies? This is purely as a result of an un-toned triceps muscle. It's so easy to tone up the triceps. And in doing so, you improve your appearance and don't feel that you have to hide your upper arms in the summer. Benefits, benefits...

Is aerobic best?

Aerobic exercise is often referred to as the best all-round exercise we can do, but opinions are now starting to change. If we focus only on aerobic conditioning, we may even take it too far. Remember earlier, in chapter 11, we discussed the osteoporotic marathon runners? The other problem with long-term endurance exercise is increased tissue acidity and greater free radical damage. The more acidic we are, as you will remember from chapter 4, the more alkaline minerals we need to replace those lost via the urine. And the more free radicals we generate, the more of those food source antioxidants we need to counteract the damage. We do not have to spend hours on the treadmill or the roads to increase our bone strength. We certainly do not want to be exercising to the extent that we stop menstruating and therefore massively reduce our progesterone levels and risk osteoporosis. If you are exercising heavily, miss two periods and are not pregnant, consider that you are overdoing it and scale back. Your skeleton will thank you for it.

The need for speed

Sprint intervals are gaining a lot of popularity. I personally love sprint intervals since they generally involve running, but you don't have to be a runner to get the benefits. You can do sprints on a bike or an elliptical trainer, or even a stair climber. In fact, an elliptical trainer will give the best all-body benefits since you are using legs and arms together, and this gives the back muscles a workout, in turn reducing the risk of vertebral crush fractures. If you are frail and/or have never exercised, please do not even consider attempting sprint intervals until you have gained a basic fitness grounding. Sprints like this are for the more advanced exerciser only, and focus more on the prevention of osteoporosis rather than its reversal.

Basically with sprint intervals you do your warm-up as normal, then start sprinting and sprint really hard for anything up to one minute. You then slow your speed down just until your breathing returns to normal (this sometimes takes up to two minutes), thereafter you repeat the sprint. Advanced athletes do 20-second sprints with 10-second recoveries. These are really hard, so I suggest that when you're first starting out, you get some advice from a personal trainer or check out some peak fitness training programme on the internet. The important thing to remember is not to do too much too soon, so if you are really out of shape please remember to start off slowly. If you were an athlete in school but haven't trained for 20 or 30 years you will NOT be able to reproduce those performances right away.

Yoga

Yoga is gaining in popularity and is widely practised by those interested in living foods, and plant-based diets in general. The two do seem to complement each other very well. Yoga has whole body benefits, and in addition to being beneficial for bone strength, particularly the more dynamic forms, it is also, as mentioned earlier, a good tool for relieving stress. It allows better tissue oxygenation, which also enables the body to utilise more nutrients, including those required for improvement of bone mineralisation. I personally have found it difficult trying to do yoga if following a book or a DVD, so attend some classes first and get to know the basics before you start doing it at home.

Yoga classes can also be very useful for those with a tendency towards depression. There is usually a very good group dynamic in a yoga class, a sympathetic instructor can help you to get the best out of your practice and you will feel supported by the other members in the class, even if initially you're not sure what you're doing. Don't get despondent if you find out that you're not very flexible; there will always be some people in yoga classes who can bend double with no apparent effort, but they've probably been doing it for years. Your flexibility will improve with time and practice. You may even finish a class having had a really good laugh, and as we know, laughing is one of the best stress busters that there is.

Other beneficial exercise opportunities

It may seem slightly odd, but even doing some household chores can help you to build bone strength. Gardening can help with back strength if you are digging and pulling out weeds. You'd also be out in the sun doing this, so you'll get some vitamin D at the same time. Even vigorous house-cleaning can have benefits, particularly going up and down stairs with a heavy vacuum cleaner. Look around you for every chance to exercise. You don't necessarily, as a friend of mine used to say, have to buy a thong and join a gym.

The keys, therefore, to exercise for the improvement of bone strength are as follows:

- Lift weights
- Do some regular sprint training if you are a more advanced exerciser
- Join a group class
- Do some yoga
- Find something you enjoy doing, which motivates and inspires you
- Do some form of exercise five times a week
- Do some exercise outdoors in the sun, so that you boost your vitamin D levels at the same time
- Get some help from a personal trainer like Alex, or gym instructor when you first start out

So is exercise the key to it all? No. It is important. But each one of the aspects discussed in this book is important. Please pay attention to all of them, but do make sure that you now get moving and stay active.

Conclusion and summary

We have seen that there are many aspects to consider in relation to the health and strength of our bones. We may even be thinking that it really is all a bit complicated and that we won't ever be able to do everything that's necessary to reverse the damage that might have been caused by our previous lifestyle habits. Don't despair. The body is always trying to do its very best. The human body is an incredible machine that is far more complex than we will ever know. We may never know exactly how one aspect works in relation to everything else. The good news, in the case of rebuilding fragile bone structure, is that we don't need to. Some readers may have heard of Warren Buffett, the billionaire who famously said that there were only two rules to making money: the first being never to lose money, and the second being never to forget rule one. We could consider prevention of osteoporosis in the same way.

Rule one, in this case, is never to lose bone. How do we lose bone? As you will have seen, we lose bone by basing the diet on meat and dairy products instead of plants. By smoking, and drinking alcohol, coffee and fizzy drinks. By not eating our greens. By acidifying our bodies with prescription medications and other harmful substances. By taking artificial hormones. By leading a sedentary lifestyle. By allowing stress to dominate our lives. By avoiding the sun at all costs. By eating a high sugar diet. By eating processed carbohydrates such as white flour, pasta, white bread and white rice, which are all stripped of their nutrients. By not taking bioavailable, wholefood-based supplements.

The good news is that those even remotely on the path of good health will not be engaging in bone-losing activities. We then just need a few more tweaks to maximise our bone-building potential, so I have incorporated a 'day in the life' section next which outlines what to do, and what to eat, in a typical bone-building day. It is stated, and widely accepted in the medical profession, that after the age of 35, women lose 1 per cent of their bone density every year. I know of sufficient people in their 60s with the bone density of the average 35 year old to appreciate that this anticipated loss cannot be considered to be normal. It is common. But what is common is not necessarily normal. There are even those who suggest that osteoporosis is genetic. If I were to believe everything the geneticists told me, I would be 'looking forward' to an old age of osteoporosis, breast cancer, high blood pressure and dementia. As Gabriel Cousens says: 'Genetics loads the gun. Environment pulls the trigger.' Our nutritional environment ultimately determines which genes are expressed, and bad genes can be permanently suppressed by good nutrition.

We absolutely are not doomed to suffer the diseases of our parents, and only 1 to 3 per cent of disease is truly attributable solely to genetics. In Europe and North America, approximately one in three women past the age of menopause will develop osteoporosis, and it will affect one in eight men in middle to older age. That is common, but it is not normal. And it absolutely does not have to be this way.

A plant-based diet and an active lifestyle ensure that we never have to lose bone, provided that it is a wholefoods diet based on greens, nutritionally dense vegetables, seeds and green juices, and not imported, hybridised, unripe and poorly mineralised fruit. This diet and this lifestyle also contain the very ingredients, as discussed in the previous chapters, which are known to support new bone formation. This is a double whammy in favour of bone protection, but, sadly, one that you will never see written up in medical texts.

A plant-based diet, together with an active lifestyle, attracts those who wish to improve every aspect of their health, vitality and wellbeing. By optimising your food and lifestyle choices you will express better health at a cellular level. This will support you not just in your bone strength, but in every other aspect of your life.

A day in the life of a bone lover

If you want to prevent osteoporosis, you're going to have to do some work. If you want to reverse it, you will have to do even more work. It will require a change in your diet, in your lifestyle, possibly in everything. But it will be totally worth it. Imagine the joy of having a healthy skeletal structure for the rest of your life. Imagine getting fitter, looking better, attaining your ideal weight and having a renewed zest for life. Imagine all of your daily tasks becoming easier because you are stronger than before. Imagine never having to worry again about the dreadful statistics surrounding this disease; knowing that it won't be likely to affect you. It is all completely achievable, and many, many people before you have managed it. Don't be put off; once you get started, it gradually becomes easier. Do it for a few weeks and it could well be that you feel so much better that you won't ever want to go back to the 'old' you again.

The plan outlined below might appear to be a massive deviation from your current daily regime. To this, I would say 'observe what the masses do, and do the opposite'; it's also known as being a contrarian. The masses are experiencing an unprecedented surge in rates of osteoporosis. The masses are becoming less fit, less mobile and less agile for every year that they are alive. The health status of the masses is failing. If you don't want the same health concerns as the masses, you will have to do what the masses don't do, or are not prepared to do. Dare to be different; dare to take responsibility.

You might not be ready to be as strict as I am in regards to my own diet and lifestyle. Don't worry. I have been upgrading my diet for so many years that it is now second nature for me to eat and live in this way. Just make a start with adding all the good things which the previous chapters have focused on. Start supplementing (Juice Plus and Bone Support are a good starting point). Gradually reduce the food items that have been proven to be detrimental. This is a marathon, not a sprint. And I'm with you all the way. Please remember that if your doctor has prescribed any specific medication for you, you must continue to take it. If, after reading this book, you decide that you no longer wish to take it, that is your decision, but do make sure that you discuss it with your doctor, and why not give him or her a copy of this book to read if you have found it useful?

On rising

Drink a glass of water with a squeeze of lemon juice in it. Add a pinch of cayenne pepper if you like, to aid your digestion.

Spray your body with Ancient Minerals Magnesium Oil and rub it in.

Make a large glass of green juice, containing added turmeric root and E3 Live liquid blue-green algae, and wheatgrass juice if you have access to it. Take Bone Support supplement, and Juice Plus fruit and vineyard blends if you are using Juice Plus. Using both the Bone Support and Juice Plus is best, but if your budget does not stretch that far, use Bone Support only. However, the two combined supplements will give you the best benefits; please use both if you can. Take your probiotics if you are using them, and add six drops of *BioSil* to your juice to boost your silicon intake, as discussed in chapter 8.

Exercise, if you are a 'morning' person. Your daily exercise can be a brisk walk for half an hour, adding hand-held weights if you can manage this. If you are fitter and a regular exerciser, go for a 30-60 minute run. Alternatively, if you are a gym member, exercise at the gym using the cardio machines or weights. A combination of cardio and weights, as outlined in chapter 12, is best for bone health. If you are an 'evening' person, do your exercises in the evening if this suits your schedule better; just make sure that you find time for them. I personally exercise after I finish work in the evening, apart from on my days off, when I run in the mornings.

Shower off the magnesium oil.

Breakfast

A good breakfast would be chia porridge with almond milk (see recipes section). If you like a warm drink with breakfast, and if you are used to tea or coffee, switch to herb teas. Avoid milk. If you have poor digestion and are using digestive enzymes, take some with your breakfast.

Morning snacks

If you are a snacker, you could have some carrot sticks, a handful of soaked almonds or some sunflower seeds. Avoid cakes, pastries and biscuits; as you have learned, they rot your bones. Ensure that you drink plenty of filtered water throughout the day. Avoid bottled water if you can, since the plastic in the thin-walled bottles leaches into the water and compromises your health. Water bottled in glass is fine; plastic is not. Avoid all fizzy carbonated drinks. Think of ways to be happy and stress-free every day, since we know that stress is highly detrimental to bone health.

Lunch

A huge green salad every day is a very healthy habit to get into, and your bones, and your whole body, will love you for it. Add some seaweed to your salad, as well as sprouted food, which you can either grow yourself or find in the produce section of supermarkets. In the USA and Canada, many supermarkets sell sprouted mung beans, radish and broccoli seeds for example. I have also seen soya bean sprouts in North America, which could have benefits for bone health. In the UK, I have seen sprouted food in Sainsbury's. Take your digestive enzymes with lunch if you are using them.

Use a home-made dressing for your salad rather than a shop-bought one if you can. Remember that practically all shop-bought dressings will be processed, contain large amounts of sugar, and are very likely to contain vinegar. Vinegar is a highly acidic molecule that is harmful to bone health. If you must use vinegar, the only 'safe' one for bones would be apple cider vinegar, which you can find in speciality stores or online. Try some of the dressings in the recipes section. I'm sure you'll find your personal favourite.

After lunch

This very much depends on where you live, and what time of the year it is. We know that vitamin D, from sunlight, is essential for bone health. If you live in the UK, you will not get any vitamin D formed in your skin between mid-October and mid-March. If you live nearer the tropics, this five-month window becomes compressed the further towards the equator you go. Do try to get out in the sun every day. It boosts the mood and it allows your body to make vitamin D. Expose as much skin as you can for 20 minutes. If you are prone to burning, go into the shade after 15 minutes. It is not necessary to use sunblock for this exposure;

indeed, if you do, you'll negate the benefits. By all means use sunblock if you are going to be out in the sun for longer than this duration. Never risk burning. If you are working indoors all day and don't get a lunch break, you're risking vitamin D deficiency. Do your best to address this. If you genuinely can't get outside, ensure that you take the Bone Support supplement. You might prefer to get your sun exposure in the morning, after breakfast; it's fine to do this.

Afternoon snacks

Low glycaemic, bone-healthy ripe fruit is fine. Try a handful of blueberries, or perhaps an apple. Ensure that any fruit you eat is as ripe as possible, since a lot of fruit can be acid-forming and add to bone loss. If you're used to having tea or coffee in the afternoon, again substitute with herb teas.

Exercise

If you are exercising after work, or if it just fits in better with your day to do it in the afternoon, take your exercise before your evening meal.

Evening meal

If you are not used to a plant-based diet, it's time to invest in some recipe books. Many vegetarian recipes contain large quantities of cheese and milk, so I recommend investing in a good vegan cookbook. For active people, one to look out for is the *Thrive Energy Cookbook*, by Brendan Brazier, a man who knows a thing or two about fitness. This book is available online, and although it is biased towards athletes, most of the recipes are accessible to everyone. Packed with 150 plant-based, nutrient-dense, wholefood recipes developed within the Thrive nutritional philosophy, the *Thrive Energy Cookbook* brings concepts that started the functional, plant-based nutrition revolution to life. Recipes are all allergen-free (or with gluten-free options) to eliminate wheat, yeast, gluten, soy, refined sugar and dairy from your diet. Another excellent book for those who wish to move towards a largely uncooked plant-based diet, is *Healthful Cuisine* by Anna-Maria Clement and Kelly Serbonich.

If your diet is currently heavily meat-based, you might not be ready for a sudden switch to plants. My advice here is simple – reduce your meat consumption to two to three times a week for the first month, and have a smaller quantity of meat for each serving. Then have it once a week for the second month. Then you'll be ready to embrace plant foods and my guess is that you won't miss meat. Take your Juice Plus vegetable capsules with your evening meal if you are using them, and your digestive enzymes if you use those.

Before bed

Ensure that you don't eat within three hours of bedtime – easy to say, possibly harder to do. I know many people who snack in front of the TV in the evenings. Watching TV late in the evening can interfere with your sleep patterns, and as you have learned in chapter 11, we need that surge of human growth hormone that occurs shortly after we fall into deep sleep. Reading, or meditation, to calm the mind prior to going to bed allows the body to go into sleep mode more naturally. Eating too close to bedtime also causes a surge in cortisol, the stress hormone that we know is bad for bones, so don't fall into this trap. If you have trouble sleeping, try a camomile or valerian tea before bed. These herbs are non-addictive and have no adverse side effects.

Your digestive system might not initially be used to the large amount of fibre present in plants, especially if you have eaten a more traditional diet for a number of years. If this is the case, ease back a bit. Have a green juice every day, but maybe your 'normal' lunch, and a bone-friendly dinner. Do this for a couple of weeks. Then start adding in the salads at lunchtime. Please do persevere, since the long-term benefits are well worth any initial digestive upset that you might associate with a change in diet. Probiotic supplements will help you with this transition, so if you find the changes uncomfortable initially, use Body Biotics and digestive enzymes to help you through.

Whenever you can during the day, think about all the things in your life that you are grateful for; this will reduce your stress levels and, as a result, reduce bone loss. Try to put aside things that stress you; remember that my father said in 100 years' time they won't matter! Take numerous deep breaths throughout the day to bring more oxygen into the body. Be the change you want to see in your body, and send your bones some love.

The recipes

All of these recipes have been chosen for their bone-building potential. Many of them are uncooked, but don't be put off; uncooked food is delicious. The lack of cooking is actually a bonus, since it makes the recipes very quick and easy to prepare – no waiting around for things to come out of the oven. The main pieces of kitchen equipment that you will need are some decent sharp knives, a blender and a food processor, plus a good juicer for your daily green juice, which I recommend having as your breakfast every day. Please see the resources section at the back of the book for information on where to find the right equipment. My website will give you further information if you're confused about anything.

Breakfasts

I like to keep breakfast very light, but I appreciate that not everyone does. Usually I suggest starting your day off with the bone-building juice that you'll find in Appendix 1. If you are an active woman or man who enjoys running and wants to maintain good bone health, try the athlete's juice below to power you through your morning training. If you're not yet doing much exercise, stick with the green juice.

If you like to eat in the morning, rather than just having green juice, I recommend chia seed porridge (see below), which will give you plenty of energy for the day.

'Blood' (athlete's juice)

Remember that if you are on a low-sugar regime for medical reasons, you will not be able to use the beetroot in this juice, but you can still use the leaves. Beetroots sold in the supermarket are often lacking their leaves, but do try to get them bunched with leaves still attached, or better still of course, grow your own. Beet leaves contain loads of calcium, iron, chlorophyll, sodium, magnesium and copper. The roots contain a powerful antioxidant called betacyanin, which lowers homocysteine levels. (High homocysteine levels are linked to increased risk of stroke, heart disease, dementia and, as you have read in chapter 9, osteoporosis.) Previous studies into beetroot and its juice have shown that it increases stamina and makes muscles more efficient, largely due to the presence of nitrites, which improve blood flow. Good news for all you runners, so, as long as you have no blood-sugar regulation problems, go ahead and make this juice. I couldn't help myself; I had to call it 'Blood', not only for its colour, but what it can do for you.

1 cucumber
5 large kale leaves
1 handful pea shoots
5 sticks celery
1 clove garlic
2.5 cm ginger
1 small beetroot, with leaves

- Run everything through a high-powered juicer, such as the Green Star Elite, and ENJOY! You may even feel as if you've had a transfusion.

Chia seed porridge

I eat this porridge after long runs. It is good for people who need to maintain their body weight, and it is a far better morning meal option than the traditional 'cereal with milk' style breakfasts that so many people have slipped into the habit of. Chia seeds are tiny, but swell up to 10 times their dry size when liquids are added, so they're very filling.

2 tablespoons chia seeds
Nut milk (see the recipe substitutions section)

- Place the chia seeds in a bowl. Add the nut milk gradually, stirring frequently. Continue to stir regularly over a 15-minute period whilst the seeds swell. Use 100 ml of milk for a thick porridge, or add more milk to give the desired consistency.
- You can add blueberries to this porridge if you like.

Soups

Soups can be enjoyed either as a starter or as a full meal, especially if consumed with my bread substitute (see the recipe substitutions section). Several of these recipes require a high-powered blender such as the Vitamix for getting the smoothest consistency, but don't worry if your blender is not as powerful – you'll still get to enjoy the lovely flavours, and your bones will get the benefits either way.

Balinese soup – an Indonesian winter warmer

1 tablespoon raw almond or rainforest nut butter
250 ml water
½ cup coconut water
2.5 cm fresh ginger root, peeled and chopped
1 clove garlic, crushed
½ to 1 fresh chilli, deseeded and chopped

1 large red pepper

Juice of 1 lime

1 tablespoon coconut oil/butter

125 g (½ cup) raw macadamia nuts, soaked

Dash of sea salt (optional)

1 handful fresh coriander

- Blend all of the ingredients except half of the coriander in a heavy-duty blender or liquidiser until smooth. Pulse in the remainder of the coriander, leaving a few green bits visible. Garnish with fresh coriander if desired.
- This soup can be served warm by placing it in serving bowls which in turn are in a container of hot water, such as the washing-up bowl. Stir carefully.

Spicy Thai soup

Juice the following:

3 carrots

3 sticks celery

1 cucumber

1 red pepper, deseeded and stalk removed

Blend the juice with:

2 handfuls spinach

1 avocado

Juice of 1 lime

3 tomatoes

2.5 cm ginger piece, grated

1 clove garlic

1 spring onion

1 tablespoon coconut oil or coconut cream powder

Sprigs of coriander (optional)

Garlic pepper to season (optional)

- This soup can be served warm if you prefer – either by placing it in a bowl in the dehydrator, stirring until warm, or placing the soup into individual bowls in a washing-up bowl containing hot water, stirring occasionally.

Max's favourite-ever Thai soup

I would be happy to have this soup every night of the week (in fact, in winter, I frequently do). It is high in antioxidants and contains lots of lovely turmeric root, which, as you have read in chapter 8, is very good for your bones. You can make it less 'green' by adding less spinach, or you can make it very green indeed by adding moringa powder. Moringa is an African leaf which is very high in nutrients that are beneficial to the whole body, including the bones. If you prefer a reddish-orange soup leave out the spinach entirely, but you'll be missing out on some important minerals if you do.

This soup serves two to four people, but I sometimes find that I can eat the whole lot if I have done a great deal of exercise beforehand. For this soup you'll need a powerful blender, such as the Vitamix. If you make the green version of the soup, please don't be put off by the colour. This is serious bone food.

350 ml water
½ cucumber
2 carrots, chopped
1 red pepper, deseeded and chopped
2 large tomatoes, quartered
1 handful fresh coriander
1-2 garlic cloves, crushed
½ stick fresh lemongrass, chopped
2.5 cm ginger root, peeled and roughly chopped
5 cm turmeric root, peeled and roughly chopped
1 tablespoon raw sesame oil

1 tablespoon tamari
Juice of 1 lime
1 handful young spinach leaves
2 fresh kaffir lime leaves
Several leaves Thai basil (holy basil)
½ teaspoon hot paprika
¼ teaspoon cayenne pepper
1 tablespoon coconut cream powder
2 teaspoons moringa leaf powder (optional)
1 teaspoon hot piri-piri seasoning
½ teaspoon Chinese five spice powder

- Blend the water, cucumber, carrots, red pepper, tomatoes, lime juice, lime leaves, lemongrass, garlic, ginger, turmeric, basil leaves, coriander, tamari and oil, starting off on a low speed setting and gradually increasing the speed to high.
- Reduce the speed to low once the soup consistency is smooth.
- Add the spinach and coconut cream powder at a low blend speed, and again gradually increase the speed until smooth.
- On a low setting, add the moringa powder (optional) and the dry spices to taste.
- This soup can be enjoyed warm or cold.

Lava soup

I think you'll love this brilliantly coloured spicy soup, which owes its fiery colour to the beetroot; I know that your bones will. Blend and enjoy!

Blend the following:
½ a beetroot, chopped
2.5 cm ginger root, chopped
350 ml filtered water or coconut water
2 tomatoes

1 red pepper
Flesh of ½-1 avocado
2 cloves garlic
½ cucumber, skin removed and chopped
½ teaspoon cayenne chilli powder
1 teaspoon turmeric powder
Lime juice, to taste

- Serve garnished with herbs of your choice.

Seaweed and miso soup

Don't be put off by the title – this warm soup tastes really good. The soup contains garlic and ginger, sources of beneficial nutrients for bone health (remember, garlic contains germanium) and will help to ward off winter bugs. Enjoy it as a light meal or use it as a starter before something more substantial. Serves one.

2-3 teaspoons dark miso paste
1 clove crushed garlic
1 teaspoon grated ginger root
2-3 teaspoons sesame oil
1 tablespoon dried seaweed
Warm water

- Place the miso paste in a soup bowl and add warm water, stirring until the paste is dissolved. Add the garlic, ginger, seaweed and oil, and top up with warm water until the bowl is almost full.
- You can garnish your soup with sprouts or have it as-is. If you want a 'hotter' taste, add a pinch of cayenne.

Watercress and cucumber soup

Chilled soups are a perfect light meal for the warmer months, and this is a lovely light and refreshing soup. Watercress is a nutritional powerhouse, and is full of minerals and vitamin K. Serves four.

¼ cup pine nuts
Flesh of 1 ripe avocado
1 cup filtered water
2 tablespoons olive oil
2 tablespoons lemon juice
2 teaspoons tamari
2 teaspoons finely grated ginger
1-2 cloves garlic, crushed
4 cups chopped cucumber
Filtered water as necessary
Pinch of sea salt (optional)
1 large handful watercress, roughly chopped
¼ cup mint leaves, chopped
2 spring onions, chopped

- In a blender, place pine nuts, one cup filtered water, avocado, olive oil, lemon juice, tamari, ginger and garlic, and blend until very smooth.
- Cut the cucumbers roughly, add to the blender and blend until smooth, adding additional water as necessary to achieve desired thickness. Season to taste with salt and black pepper (optional).
- Add watercress, mint and spring onions and blend until mixed, but with little bits of the herbs still visible.
- Serve chilled, and garnish with a small sprig of watercress or mint.

'Complete Meal' green energy soup

Blend together the following:

Chopped cucumber
Chopped celery
Chopped broccoli, including the stem
Red onion
Chopped fresh herbs (I use parsley, dill and basil)
Diced avocado
Lemon juice
1-2 cups of bone-building green juice (see Appendix 1)
Crushed garlic

Broccoli and Turmeric Soup

2 cups water
4 cups chopped broccoli
1 red pepper
2 red onions
2 sticks celery, chopped
1 medium avocado
1 tablespoon tamari
2.5 cm turmeric root, peeled
2.5 cm ginger root, peeled
1 clove garlic

- Warm the water to hand-hot by placing in a bain-marie or on a low heat. Add broccoli and warm for five minutes. Transfer the broccoli and water to a blender, add the other ingredients and blend until smooth.
- Serve warm. Serves four.

Creamy asparagus soup

12-15 asparagus spears, chopped
5 large vine-ripened tomatoes, roughly chopped
1 cup fresh parsley
3 cloves garlic
½ cup fresh dill
2 spring onions, chopped
1 red or yellow pepper, chopped
Juice of 1 lemon
2 teaspoons tamari
1 tablespoon coconut cream powder or 3-oz coconut cream block, dissolved in water
Water to blend

- Blend all ingredients until a smooth consistency is reached, adding a little water if the mixture is too thick.
- Blend in the coconut cream powder (or dissolved block coconut) at the end.
- Can be served warm or cold, unless using coconut block, which necessitates warming.

Creamy mushroom soup

1 cup shiitake mushrooms with stems removed
1-2 tablespoons raw almond butter (you'll find this in good independent health food stores or online)
2 cups almond milk (shop-bought, or preferably home-made)
½ red onion, chopped
½ cup fresh parsley
3 sticks celery, chopped
1 handful spinach, chopped
½ tablespoon sesame oil
1 teaspoon tamari or Bragg's Liquid Aminos

- Blend the mushrooms, almond butter and almond milk in a blender. Try to get a smooth consistency. Add the onion, parsley and tamari and blend again, but leaving little bits for a flavour burst. Pour the soup into bowls.
- In another bowl, mix the finely chopped celery with the spinach and sesame oil. Use to garnish the soup.
- This soup can be served cold or warm. If serving warm, add the garnish after heating.

Chlorophyll soup

1 organic avocado (skin and stone removed)
1 organic courgette
¼ large cucumber
3 organic celery sticks
1 small fennel bulb
1 large handful organic spinach
1 large handful organic watercress
1 large clove garlic (crushed)
Juice of ½ lemon
Several fresh basil leaves
Small handful sunflower sprouts (optional)
1 dessertspoon raw tahini
1 tablespoon Udo's Choice oil, olive oil or sesame oil
2 or more tablespoons filtered water

- Put all ingredients in a large blender or food processor and combine well. Add water to reach your desired consistency.
- For a spicier taste, try adding some dried or fresh red chillies. To go a bit more exotic, add Nasi Kuning, an Indonesian combination of coconut and spices. You can also sprinkle hemp seeds on top for a heavier meal.
- This soup feeds two very hungry people. It contains an excellent balance of minerals and is very alkalising. It is high in calcium

and magnesium. The celery provides organic sodium so this is a good meal after heavy exercise.

- As with all of the other blended soups in this section, the soup can be warmed in winter by putting serving bowls into a washing-up bowl with hot water in it, pouring the soup into the bowls and stirring every five minutes for 15 to 20 minutes. This ensures none of the heat-sensitive nutrients are destroyed.

Salads, pâtés and wraps

Salads can be enjoyed at any time of day, and at any time of year. They can be considered to be a main course as well, particularly the more 'dense' salads that contain soaked nuts and seeds.

These salad ideas really are just a starting point. Once you get into the habit of having salads regularly, you can experiment by adding some of the sprouted foods such as quinoa and amaranth (small grains, see chapter 4), mung beans, lentils and chick peas to make them into a heartier and more filling meal. Remember that the pâtés are an excellent accompaniment to many salads, and by using them together you'll have a main meal.

Kale, parsley and avocado salad

Kale and parsley are rich in bone-building minerals and vitamin C. Vitamin K, present in the greens, is fat-soluble, and the healthy fats in the olive oil and avocado will help you to absorb it. The lemon juice is alkalising and gives you extra vitamin C, as does the red pepper. The sesame seeds are a good source of calcium, and hemp seeds contain plenty of minerals.

6-8 handfuls of green curly kale, chopped up small and with the tough stalks removed
¼ cup chopped fresh parsley
1 red bell pepper, diced

1 ripe avocado, diced
2 tablespoons extra virgin olive oil
Pinch Celtic sea salt, or a dash of tamari or Bragg's Liquid Aminos
Juice of 1 lemon
2 tablespoons sesame seeds or hemp seeds

- In a large bowl, massage the kale, olive oil and salt (or tamari or Bragg's Liquid Aminos) together until the kale leaves look slightly wilted.
- Add the avocado, red pepper, parsley and lemon juice and mix in well.
- Sprinkle the sesame or hemp seeds on top and serve.
- Serves two.

Sprouty summer salad

This is a great summer recipe, and something that I eat every day, regardless of the season. Modify any ingredients to your own personal taste, and buy organic whenever you can. Serves two.

100 g wild rocket
100 g baby leaf spinach
100 g watercress
50 g pea shoots
4 tablespoons mung bean sprouts
4 tablespoons buckwheat sprouts (optional)
50 g alfalfa, red clover or sango radish sprouts, rinsed (or a mixture of all three)
A few mint leaves
Juice of 1 lemon
1 large garlic clove, crushed
1 sprig parsley
1 medium fully ripe avocado, diced

1 red pepper, diced
1-2 tablespoons raw sesame or flax oil

- Chop all the greens in a large bowl.
- Add the sprouts, red pepper, garlic and avocado.
- Combine everything with the sesame oil and lemon juice and mix well.
- Enjoy for lunch in the sun, or dinner after a great day doing what you love best.

Summer fruit and leaf salad

Watermelon and tomatoes are low-sugar fruits which give you plenty of lycopene, a phytonutrient that helps you to avoid sunburn; important for when you're out there topping up your vitamin D levels (see chapter 9). Watercress is loaded with vitamin K for your bones.

Watermelon, diced into 2.5-cm cubes
1 red or pink grapefruit, divided into segments and pith removed
2-3 tomatoes, sliced
1 handful of watercress per person
Alfalfa sprouts and pomegranate to garnish

- Place one slice of tomato in four or five places on the perimeter of a plate (this is great if you have square plates – one at each corner). On top of each slice, place a segment of grapefruit and a cube of watermelon.
- Pile up some watercress in the centre of the plate.
- Finish off with a sprinkling of alfalfa sprouts and scatter some pomegranate seeds over the whole. I just eat mine as-is, but if you fancy a dressing with it, keep it light and citrus-y, perhaps with a tang of miso.

An Asian-flavoured appetiser

It's amazing what you can do with a few ingredients and a bit of spice. I haven't even given this particular first course a name yet, so if you can come up with one, please let me know. Seaweed makes an appearance here again for its mineral content. Serves four as a first course.

125 g raw cashews or macadamia nuts
1 large tomato
1 tablespoon raw sesame oil
2 tablespoons sesame seeds or hemp seeds
2.5 cm piece of ginger, finely grated
½ a spring onion (scallion)
½ teaspoon Chinese five-spice powder
A few sprigs of coriander (cilantro) (optional)
1 tablespoon raw nori sprinkles (I use Clearspring brand)
1 tablespoon ground flax seed
4 pak choi leaves

- Blend everything except the pak choi leaves in a food processor, but make sure the nuts end up with a chopped consistency, not totally broken down.
- Lay four pak choi leaves on a plate and use the nut and seed mixture to 'fill' the leaves. If the mixture is a little watery, add a bit more flax powder.
- Feel free to add more spices if you prefer it hotter.

Sprouted buckwheat tabbouleh

Tabbouleh, a traditional Middle Eastern recipe, generally involves the use of bulghur wheat. This recipe contains gluten-free sprouted buckwheat instead. The recipe comes from Judy Barber's book, *Good Raw Food Recipes*, an excellent book full of high-nutrient density plant-based recipes.

2 cups buckwheat, soaked overnight and sprouted for two days
½ cup finely chopped parsley
½ cup chopped cucumber
1 finely chopped red pepper
¼ cup chopped mild onion
Chopped mint (optional)
2 tablespoons lemon juice
2 tablespoons cold-pressed olive oil
Powdered sea vegetables or tamari to taste

- Combine all ingredients in a large bowl and serve.

Nori wraps

These wraps are quite possibly my all-time favourite food. Incredibly filling and sustaining, I bet you can't eat more than three! They are loaded with goodness and nori is excellent for bone health, due to its mineral content, as well as feeding the thyroid, due to its high iodine content.

Serves two (three wraps each; reduce the quantities accordingly for smaller appetites).

6 raw nori sheets
2 large handfuls spinach
2 large handfuls rocket
1 handful watercress
½ cup buckwheat sprouts
½ cup mung bean sprouts
2 tablespoons small green sprouts, for example alfalfa, sango radish, broccoli
½ small head broccoli
2 large tomatoes, chopped
1 medium avocado, diced
1 red pepper, finely chopped (optional)

1-2 cloves garlic, crushed
Juice of 1 lemon
2 tablespoons pine nuts
4-6 sun-dried tomatoes in oil, chopped
2 tablespoons raw pesto (see recipe below)

- Chop the salad leaves with kitchen scissors. Add all the remaining ingredients except the nori and stir well.
- Spread out a nori sheet and place the salad mixture across the lower part of the sheet.
- Fold the sides in so the mixture can't escape, and roll the sheet up. Seal the long end by wetting it with a little water, and press down.
- You can cut your nori wrap with a very sharp knife to make sushi rolls, but I prefer to just eat it as it is.
- Caution: it can get a bit messy!

Hey pesto!

I love pesto. This recipe came about because I have, for a number of years, occasionally been buying a very special raw vegan Italian pesto in a jar. It's totally delicious, but somewhat expensive, and the salt content isn't great for bone health. A recent experiment in the kitchen has brought forward the following green treat. I hope you love it too!

Good quality cold-pressed olive oil
150 g pine nuts, unroasted cashews, or a combination of both
100-150 g fresh basil leaves
Juice of 1 lemon
2 cloves crushed garlic
Pinch of sea salt, to taste

- Combine all ingredients in a blender on a low speed setting.

Process until smooth. Add more oil or lemon juice for a thinner consistency if required.

- This pesto makes a fantastic addition to a summer salad. It will keep for a few days in the fridge, but might not last that long because it's so yummy it's likely to be eaten straight away!

Basic greens and avocado salad

So very easy and fast to make, this salad is great for its mineral content and healthy fats. Serves two to three.

4 handfuls of a mixture of green leaves, including watercress, wild rocket, coriander and spinach
2 large avocados, stone and skin removed, diced
10-20 pitted raw black olives (avoid those which are chemically preserved and bottled in vinegar)
Juice of 1 lemon
Drizzle of cold-pressed olive oil

- Chop the salad leaves and make them into a bed on which to mix the other ingredients together.

Almond romaine salad

1 head romaine lettuce, torn into small pieces
1 handful young spinach leaves, torn into small pieces
2 spring onions, chopped
1 cup (250 g) raw almonds, soaked overnight and brown skins removed
3 tablespoons lemon juice
3 tablespoons extra virgin olive oil
1 teaspoon celery seasoning

- Combine everything in a bowl.

- Add more lemon for a sharper flavour, or substitute with lime juice for a different citrus tang.

Orange and ginger sprouts

2 teaspoons fresh grated ginger
Juice of 2 large oranges
100 g (1 bag) organic macadamia nuts, previously soaked for three or more hours
Alfalfa sprouts, or other small-leafed sprouts such as broccoli, red clover or radish

- Blend the orange juice, soaked macadamias and ginger in a blender or liquidiser until smooth.
- Pour over alfalfa sprouts and serve.

Rainbow shredded veggies

It's good to eat all the colours of the rainbow, and this fantastic mix will get you there. Cabbage is great for bone health, and this simple salad/coleslaw will really get your antioxidant levels buzzing.

Half a purple cabbage
1 head broccoli
2 red peppers, stem and seeds removed
2 orange peppers, stem and seeds removed
1 yellow or red onion
4 small purple heirloom carrots, or 2 medium orange carrots if heirloom varieties are not available
1 raw beetroot
2 parsnips
4 tablespoons lemon juice
1 tablespoon tamari or Bragg's Liquid Aminos

3 tablespoons raw sesame oil (add more if needed)
1-2 garlic cloves, crushed
1-2 teaspoons seaweed powder to taste

- Shred the cabbage, onion, broccoli, carrots, peppers, parsnips and beetroot in a food processor. Transfer the mixture to a large bowl.
- Mix the lemon juice, sesame oil, garlic and tamari together. Pour over the shredded vegetables and mix well.
- Add the seaweed powder according to taste.

Tahini and miso spread and sauce

Tahini is pulped sesame paste, and makes a frequent appearance in Middle Eastern recipes. The following three recipes come from my friend and colleague Judy Barber, author of the excellent book *Good Raw Food Recipes* (www.goodrawfoodrecipes.com). Judy designs the menus for the retreats and residential weekends which we run together (see www.rawfoodretreat.eu for more information).

You barely need a recipe for this spread. The ingredients are simply tahini and the slightly salty fermented soybean paste called miso, which is also good for bone health. Make sure you use unpasteurised miso, which is easier to find in health food shops than in regular shops. Unpasteurised miso provides helpful probiotics (see chapter 10).

Mix a quarter cup of miso with one and a half cups of tahini in a bowl. You can use this mixture as a spread on crackers or in raw wraps such as lettuce leaf wraps, along with other fillings. For a creamy sauce to pour over chopped salad vegetables, stir in one to one and a half cups of water. I never tire of this delicious sauce and it's surprising how interesting it tastes from such a simple – and quick – recipe.

Cucumber and tahini pâté

By drinking green vegetable juice (see appendix 1) you do your bones a favour and also have vegetable fibres/pulp to hand. Cucumber fibres are the softest and make a great pâté ingredient. You can use them to thicken a pâté. For example, mix cucumber fibres and tahini roughly 50/50 and mix in a little miso to taste. Depending on your juicer, you may need to add a little cucumber juice to soften the pâté. For variety, add finely chopped herbs. Serve sprinkled with chopped herbs and drizzled with cold-pressed olive oil.

Pumpkin seed pesto

Pumpkin seeds are another bone-friendly seed, rich in zinc (see chapter 8). In this recipe pumpkin seeds replace the traditional pine nuts that can be so very expensive. For optimum nutrition and digestibility it is important to soak the pumpkin seeds for a few hours beforehand.

- In a food processor mix all of the following to a smooth paste:

½ cup soaked pumpkin seeds
¼ cup water
The juice of ½ lemon
Optional: splashes of tamari or Bragg's Liquid Aminos to taste
A medium clove of garlic
¼ cup of cold-pressed olive oil

- Separately, chop a medium-sized bunch of fresh basil leaves very finely. Stir them into the pumpkin seed mixture or pulse for a second.
- Serve the pesto stirred into pasta, preferably into 'courgette pasta' made from thin shavings of courgette cut with a potato peeler.

Humous

1 tablespoon raw tahini
1 cup sprouted chick peas, or substitute cooked chick peas if you haven't taken up sprouting yet
1 large clove garlic, crushed
Juice of 2 lemons
1 tablespoon cold-pressed olive oil
Small amount filtered water
2 sprigs fresh parsley, or small handful fresh coriander

- Blend all the ingredients together.
- Use as a dip for vegetables or a salad dressing.

Salad dressings

What do you put on your salads? This is a question I am often asked, particularly when people realise that I have a total aversion to vinegar and to any shop-bought salad dressing. I think it's a throwback to my childhood when I was presented with a glass jar of some horrible processed gloopy liquid that smelt awful, that was supposed to make the salad 'taste nice'. Urgh! I'm personally quite happy to munch through lots of green leaves on their own with no salad dressing at all, but I appreciate that not everyone is of the same disposition. Here are a few options for salad dressings that even I like, so they must be good. As you'll see, there's no vinegar anywhere. You will have read in chapter 4 that vinegar is an acidic molecule, so we will be doing our bones a great favour by not using it. By avoiding vinegar, you'll let the real flavour of the food itself shine through.

Really basic dressing

½ cup lemon juice
½ cup extra virgin olive oil

1 clove garlic, crushed
Pinch of cayenne pepper
Pinch of ground cumin
Fresh or dried herbs (parsley and oregano work well)

- Shake the ingredients together in a lidded jar.
- Keep refrigerated.

Lemon tahini dressing

1 tablespoon raw tahini
1 large clove garlic, crushed
Juice of 2 lemons
Small amount filtered water
2 sprigs fresh parsley, or small handful fresh coriander

- Blend all the ingredients together. Use as a dip for vegetables or a salad dressing.

Tomato and olive dressing

20 black olives, stones removed
2 organic tomatoes

- Blend the tomatoes and olives together and use as a salad dressing.
- If you want a really amazing coloured dressing of a slightly thicker consistency, add two teaspoons of raw tahini.

Asian-style dressing

This dressing is fabulous with Chinese-style vegetables. It contains tahini, which is good for bone health, and ginger, the benefits of which you have read about in chapter 9. You can substitute ginger for turmeric if you like. It does contain honey, and as we know, honey is high in sugar. I therefore recommend that you either substitute the honey for liquid stevia to get the sweetness, or use the dressing less frequently than the other types. This recipe makes a large amount of dressing, so reduce the quantities for your personal requirements if you need to.

1 cup (250 g) raw tahini
1½ cups filtered water
3 tablespoons sesame oil
3 tablespoons flax oil
¾ cup tamari or Bragg's Liquid Aminos
3 tablespoons grated ginger or turmeric root
3 spring onions, finely chopped
2-3 cloves garlic, crushed
2 tablespoons honey, or substitute with a few drops of liquid stevia or 2 pinches powdered stevia
¾ teaspoon Chinese five-spice powder
½ teaspoon cayenne pepper
½ teaspoon cumin powder

- Blend all ingredients together in a food processor or blender.

Creamy pine nut dressing

1 cup pine nuts or sunflower seeds, soaked
½ cup almonds, soaked and skins removed
2 cups filtered water
2 cloves garlic
½ teaspoon dried rosemary or oregano
2-3 tablespoons Bragg's Liquid Aminos or tamari

- Blend all ingredients together until smooth.
- Chill before serving.

Watercress dressing

1 large avocado
1 bunch watercress
1 cucumber
Juice of 1 lemon
2 cloves garlic, crushed
1 piece dried seaweed, for example dulse, rinsed to remove excess salt

- Blend all ingredients until smooth.

Special flax seed dressing

Flax seeds are a great source of essential fatty acids. They are anti-inflammatory and are good for joint pain.

2 tablespoons flax seeds, soaked for four to five hours
½ cup sunflower seeds, soaked for five hours, rinsed and drained
2 cloves garlic, crushed
1 tablespoon fresh dill
2 tablespoons fresh lemon juice
Tamari or Bragg's Liquid Aminos, to taste
2 cups chopped cucumber
¼-½ cup filtered water

- Blend the soaked seeds, garlic, herbs, lemon juice and tamari/ Bragg's Liquid Aminos, adding water slowly until a smooth consistency is reached.
- Slowly add the cucumber pieces and blend until smooth.
- Adjust the consistency with water as required. Season to taste.

Avocado-based dipping sauce

This sauce can be used as a salad dressing or for dipping crudités. It has a thicker consistency than the other dressings above.

1 avocado
3 tomatoes
1 medium carrot
1 stick celery
4 sun-dried tomatoes
½ teaspoon kelp
1 medjool date
¼ onion or 3 spring onions
1 teaspoon tamari
1 teaspoon olive oil

- Blend all the ingredients together.

Red pepper and pine nut sauce

2 red peppers
6 sun-dried tomatoes (preferably in oil, no vinegar)
6-8 cherry tomatoes
½ cup pine nuts
½ apple, cored
1 teaspoon dried mixed herbs
1 teaspoon garlic granules
¼ teaspoon chilli

- Blend all the ingredients together.

Main courses

Spinach and garlic stuffed mushrooms

These lovely stuffed mushrooms can be used as a main course or a side dish. The greens contain lots of lovely bone-building minerals, and certain types of mushrooms contain vitamin D. You might be familiar with the well-used phrase, 'Life's too short to stuff a mushroom'. Not when they taste like this it isn't!

6-8 mushrooms (either large portabella mushrooms or slightly smaller ones depending on your preference)

Marinade:
1 cup of olive oil (add more oil and tamari if needed)
1 tablespoon tamari
3 garlic cloves, crushed
Juice of ½ lemon
Pinch of Himalayan salt (optional)

Stuffing:
½ bag spinach (approx 1 cup, close-packed)
100 g bag pine nuts
1 garlic clove
1 handful fresh basil
A little fresh thyme
1 tablespoon tamari
Pinch of Himalayan salt

- Peel the mushrooms and remove stalks, keeping mushrooms whole. Marinate for a few hours, stirring occasionally until all are well coated.
- Put all stuffing ingredients into a food processor and process until the mixture forms a fairly thick, smooth consistency, adding a little water as necessary.

- Put spoonfuls of the spinach stuffing mix into each mushroom and dehydrate for a few hours until mushrooms are warm and soft. Serve while the mushrooms are still warm.

Vegetable curry

I love spicy food, and as we've learned, it can be very good for our bone health, with the recognised benefits of turmeric root. This is a good warming winter recipe when made in the dehydrator. This recipe comes courtesy of the Hippocrates Health Institute. You can substitute other vegetables if you like. I have found that this recipe works very well when using sweet potato.

1 cup diced red pepper
1 cup quartered mushrooms
1 cup small broccoli florets
1 cup small cauliflower florets
1 cup halved and sliced courgette
½ cup chopped fresh coriander
1 cup halved and sliced carrot
2 spring onions, sliced diagonally

Dressing

½ cup Hippocrates' House Dressing (see below)
½ cup chopped red pepper
¼ cup spring onions
1 teaspoon curry powder, garam masala, or dried turmeric
¼ cup water
1 tablespoon raw sesame oil, or other oil
Dash of liquid stevia (optional)

Hippocrates House Dressing

1 cup high-quality oil
2¼ tablespoons fresh lemon juice

2½ tablespoons Bragg's Liquid Aminos or Nama Shoyu
2 cloves garlic
2 teaspoons ground mustard seed
¼ teaspoon cayenne pepper

- Combine the vegetables in a large bowl.
- Blend the dressing ingredients. Pour over the vegetables and mix in thoroughly – you can do this with your hands if you like.
- Leave to stand for 30 minutes before serving. If you like, you can spread the mixture on two dehydrator trays and dehydrate at 105ºF for 30-60 minutes. This softens the vegetables and warms the curry – heaven!

Carrot and macadamia pâté

Carrots contain not just beta carotene but over 40 other carotenoid pigments, which act as powerful antioxidants. You can substitute the macadamia nuts for sunflower seeds if you prefer a slightly lighter consistency. Serves four as a starter/appetiser, or two as a main course.

4 large carrots, grated
30 g ginger, grated
100-125 g raw macadamia nuts, soaked overnight
1-2 tablespoons sesame oil
1 teaspoon Chinese five-spice powder
Garlic pepper, to taste

- Place all the ingredients in a blender and blend to a smooth consistency. Season with garlic pepper to your own taste preference.
- Use the pâté as it is, or mould it if you prefer. It's a great accompaniment to salad greens.

Fiery sweet potatoes

This hot and spicy dish is an excellent substitute for 'normal' potatoes. Sweet potatoes contain half the sugar and four times the mineral content of regular white potatoes, and are a better option than cooked white potatoes, which can increase tissue acidity and promote inflammation.

1-2 tablespoons olive oil
2 teaspoons Tamari or Nama Shoyu (raw soy sauce)
1 tablespoon minced garlic
1 tablespoon minced ginger root
½ teaspoon dried red chilli, or ½ a fresh red chilli
½ teaspoon cayenne pepper
1-2 tablespoons water if needed
3 cups grated sweet potatoes

- In a small bowl or blender whisk the oil, tamari, garlic, ginger and cayenne. Add additional water if needed to achieve the desired consistency.
- Place sweet potatoes in a bowl and pour dressing over, stirring in before serving.
- This is great as an accompaniment to salad, or on its own as a filling snack or meal in its own right.

Sunny stuffed peppers

2 cups sunflower seeds, soaked 12 hours and sprouted for a further 24 hours
1 cup chick pea sprouts
½ red pepper, deseeded and sliced
1 clove garlic, crushed
Juice of ½ lemon
1 dessertspoon raw tahini
1 organic tomato

1 handful fresh coriander
4 red or orange peppers, halved lengthways and deseeded

- Blend all the ingredients except the halved peppers until smooth. Stuff the mixture into the peppers.
- Serve on a bed of mixed green leaves.

Mediterranean stuffed red peppers

1 organic avocado, skin and stone removed
20 stoned raw black olives
½ packet sun-dried tomatoes, soaked and drained
1 clove garlic, crushed
1 dessertspoon raw tahini
Juice of ½ lemon
Handful fresh coriander
20 sunflower sprouts (optional)
2 large Ramiro red peppers (the pointed ones)
Alfalfa sprouts to garnish

- Put everything except the last two ingredients in a blender or food processor and blend until smooth.
- Cut the peppers along one long side only, remove the seeds.
- Fill the peppers with the mixture, finishing off with alfalfa sprouts and some small cubes of fresh avocado if desired.
- Serve on a bed of mixed green leaves.

Raw fry

$^{2}/_{3}$ block creamed coconut
Filtered water
1 handful fresh coriander
½ a red chilli, deseeded
Juice of 2 limes

1 tablespoon raw organic sesame oil
2 teaspoons grated fresh ginger
1 large garlic clove, crushed
1 packet exotic vegetables (you will find these as a 'do it yourself' stir-fry in most supermarkets. Discard the packet of sauce that is often provided with the vegetables and use this recipe instead.)

- Firstly make the coconut milk. Chop the creamed coconut into small pieces, and add enough warm (not hot) water to make a fairly thick sauce. Stir well until all coconut is dissolved.
- Put into a blender with all other ingredients except the exotic vegetables. Process until a smooth sauce is made. This should smell fantastic!
- Put the exotic vegetable mixture into bowls, pour sauce over and serve.
- Other vegetables can be used – try including broccoli, bean sprouts, mushrooms; anything you like really. For extra warmth on a cold day, mix a few raw and soaked nuts in with the vegetables.

Spaghetti bolognese

Here is a 'Love your Bones' version of the Italian classic. Meat-free, gluten-free, mineral-dense and guilt-free – all the things that the original is not.

For the pasta

4 large courgettes, spiralised. A spiraliser is a wonderful piece of kitchen equipment that makes ribbon-like lengths of vegetables. If you don't have one or can't find one online, you can shave the courgette into lengths with a potato peeler instead.

For the bolognese sauce
5 large tomatoes
1 pack sun-dried tomatoes, soaked and rinsed
1-2 cloves garlic
Juice of 2 lemons
Several basil leaves
20 stoned olives, or ½ jar olive paste

- Blend all of the sauce ingredients until smooth. If you are avoiding tomatoes, you can substitute the tomatoes with two medium-sized red peppers, and substitute the sun-dried tomatoes with half a cup of soaked sunflower seeds.
- Place the spiralised or shaved courgettes into a large serving dish and pour the sauce on top.

Pine nut burgers

For people who like heavier foods, these meat-free 'burgers' are ideal. Even people who like typical fast-food hamburgers seem to like these, and of course they are streets apart from a health perspective. This recipe requires a dehydrator for best results, but don't panic if you haven't got one. You can use the top oven on the lowest setting and leave the door slightly open, or if you have an Aga, you can make the burgers using the warming oven.

1 cup pine nuts
1 cup pecan nuts
2 carrots, grated
1 cup each of fresh basil, mint and parsley, finely chopped
1 dessertspoon olive oil
Small pinch sea salt or ground seaweed

- Put the pecan nuts in a food processor first and process until finely chopped. Add the remainder of the ingredients and process until the mixture starts to stick together.

- Spread the mixture ¼-inch thick onto a dehydrator tray, or roll into balls and press into burger shapes. If the mixture is too wet just put spoonfuls onto the tray and press down flat. Dehydrate at 100-118ºF for a few hours, then turn and dehydrate for a few more hours or overnight, depending on thickness of burger.
- If you're using the top oven or Aga, make the burgers in the evening, leave them in the oven overnight and test the next day to ensure they're dry enough. Enjoy with salad.

Pumpkin seed and walnut loaf

2 cups pumpkin seeds, soaked for six to eight hours
2 cups walnuts, soaked overnight
1 cup carrot, chopped
1 cup red pepper, deseeded and chopped
1 cup onion, diced
1 cup parsley, chopped
1 cup dried mushrooms
2 cloves garlic, crushed
1 tablespoon raw tahini (optional)
Sprig of parsley to garnish

- Process the pumpkin seeds, walnuts and carrot in a food processor until smooth. Remove and place in a bowl.
- Pulse the remaining ingredients except the parsley together in a food processor until they are of a chunky consistency. Place in the bowl with the pumpkin seed mixture and combine thoroughly.
- Place on a serving dish and mould into the desired shape. Garnish with parsley.

Mock tuna

Do you enjoy tuna salads? Try this 'mock' tuna instead; I think you'll be a convert.

3 cups walnuts, soaked for 12 hours then drained
3 cups carrots
1 medium onion
1 cup chopped celery
½ cup parsley, chopped
¼ cup fresh tarragon
¼ cup fresh dill
3 cloves garlic, crushed
Juice of 2 lemons
Tamari or Bragg's Liquid Aminos, to taste
Dehydrated vegetables, optional

- Process the walnuts and carrots in a food processor or through a juicer with the blank screen attachment.
- Pulse the garlic, onion, celery and herbs in a food processor until coarsely chopped.
- Place all ingredients in a bowl and mix until consistent.
- Form into the desired shape on a serving dish, and garnish with parsley, herbs or other greens.

Cooked options

Not everyone wants to eat uncooked food the whole time. Whilst cooking your food can contribute to more acidity in the body (see chapter 4), the recipes below will help those who are just starting off on their bone-loving path. Now that you have read that avoiding animal protein (meat, fish, dairy and eggs) is important for bone health, you might be wondering what on earth you can actually eat (apart from salads of course). I hope that you'll enjoy these three recipes and realise that a plant-based diet is certainly not consistent with deprivation.

Baked sweet potatoes with rosemary

This filling dish is ideal on a cold day, and it's so simple because there are only four ingredients. It's another great recipe for those who feel they are not ready to leave roast potatoes behind. I think you may be converted once you taste these.

3 sweet potatoes
1 tablespoon coconut oil, melted
6 cloves garlic, peeled
4 sprigs rosemary

- Pre-heat the oven to 350ºF (180ºC, gas mark 4).
- Scrub the sweet potatoes but do not peel them. Dice into bite-sized chunks and place in a heatproof lidded dish.
- Remove the rosemary leaves from the woody stem and discard the stem.
- Add the coconut oil, whole garlic cloves and rosemary to the sweet potatoes and stir in.
- Bake for approx 30 minutes or until the sweet potatoes become soft.

Chick pea curry

This curry contains turmeric, which is good for bone health (see chapter 9). Make it as hot and spicy as you like. Serves two.

1 small onion
2 large handfuls spinach
½-1 can chickpeas, rinsed and drained, or 1 cup sprouted chickpeas (preferable)

¼ block coconut cream, dissolved in warm water, or 1 tablespoon coconut cream powder
1 teaspoon garam masala
¾ teaspoon ground turmeric
½ teaspoon ground cumin
2 teaspoons coconut oil
Water as needed

- Heat the coconut oil in a frying pan. Add the onion and fry on a low heat until the onion becomes clear but not brown.
- Add the chickpeas, coconut cream, spinach, garlic and spices and simmer until the spinach wilts and the curry is warmed through. Add a little extra water if needed.
- Serve either with steamed quinoa, sprouted black rice or steamed wholegrain rice.

Lentil and vegetable casserole

1 tablespoon coconut oil
1 onion, finely chopped
3 garlic cloves, sliced
1 teaspoon smoked paprika
½ teaspoon ground cumin
1 tablespoon dried thyme
3 medium carrots, sliced (about 200g)
2 medium sticks celery, finely sliced (about 120g)
1 red pepper, deseeded and chopped
1 yellow pepper, deseeded and chopped
20 peeled cherry tomatoes
250 ml vegetable stock cube (choose one that is low in salt)
2 courgettes, sliced thickly (about 300 g)
2 sprigs fresh thyme
250 g (1 cup) cooked or sprouted lentils

- Heat the coconut oil in a large, heavy-based pan. Add the onions and cook gently for five to 10 minutes until softened.
- Add the garlic, spices, dried thyme, carrots, celery and peppers and cook for five minutes.
- Add the tomatoes, stock, courgettes and fresh thyme and cook for 20 to 25 minutes.
- Take out the thyme sprigs. Stir in the lentils and bring back to a simmer.
- Serve with steamed quinoa or wild black rice.

Substitutions for common processed foods

It's a potential problem when you're on a bone-loving routine, since we are all surrounded by salt- and sugar-laden unhealthy snack foods and things that we know we now need to avoid, such as milk and cheese. Here are a few ideas for healthy snacks, giving alternatives to biscuits, crisps (potato chips for my North American readers), desserts and dairy products. Make the switch; your bones will really appreciate you for it.

Sprouted buckwheat biscuits

What about biscuits? Here is an alternative for everyone who's wondering how to substitute something for those unhealthy, fat- and sugar-laden, addictive sweet biscuits that reduce bone health and strength. Why not try them with a cup of herb tea?

250 g (1 cup) raw buckwheat, soaked overnight, rinsed and sprouted for one day
½ cup desiccated coconut
1 cup sunflower seeds, soaked one to two hours and drained
2 teaspoons maca powder
2 teaspoon lucuma powder
1 teaspoon vanilla powder

1 teaspoon mixed spice
Stevia for sweetness (optional)

- Put all the ingredients into a food processor and mix in short bursts, using a spatula to help move the mixture in between bursts, since it is fairly dry.
- Place tablespoon-sized amounts onto the dehydrator sheets and with a wet knife and wet hands shape each portion into flat round 'biscuits'. Handle the biscuits as little as possible otherwise they can end up being quite hard.
- Dehydrate for a few hours and lift each one individually onto a tray without a sheet and dehydrate for a further eight hours or more. Dehydrate overnight if possible so that they become very crumbly.

Carob chia mousse

This recipe is ideal for anyone who normally likes a stodgy dessert. It's a useful option to substitute for processed sweet mousses that contain large amounts of unhealthy fat and sugar.

Blend the following:

½ avocado
½ banana
1 teaspoon raw carob powder
½ cup soaked almonds
2 teaspoons chia seeds
1 tablespoon ground almonds (optional)
Tiny drop of water

- Blend all the ingredients together.
- Place in ramekin dishes and chill for half an hour before serving.

Bread

One of the food items many of us might miss on a bone-loving routine is bread. After all, who wouldn't confess to enjoying a big bowl of hot soup and a door-wedge of bread on a cold day? And what about sandwiches? Here is my bone-loving bread recipe. It can be used for sandwiches, wraps, dunking into soups and is a great, grain-free substitute for the 'regular' bread that many people might have a problem with in respect of gluten, and which, in turn, does your bones no favours.

3 cups sweetcorn
2-2½ cups chopped carrots
3 small courgettes (zucchini)
1 red pepper
7 sun-dried tomatoes, soaked
½ cup sprouted flax powder
¼ cup olive oil
1½ teaspoon turmeric
2 teaspoons lemon and thyme seasoning
1 teaspoon medium curry powder
1 tablespoon tamari
3 cloves garlic, crushed
1 teaspoon hot paprika
Juice of ½ lemon
Any fresh herbs of your choice (oregano is good in this recipe)

- Process everything in a food processor until it is a relatively smooth paste. Spread out evenly on two dehydrator sheets to about 1 cm thickness.
- Dehydrate at 105ºF for about eight hours, or overnight. Flip the bread over, remove the Teflex sheet and dehydrate for a further five to six hours, or until desired degree of dryness is obtained.
- This bread is flexible and pliable enough to make wraps without

breaking. Enjoy it in a sandwich with salad filling, or with a blended soup, such as one of those in this book.

Nori crackers

Everyone who has tried these crackers loves them. They are great as a quick snack and fantastic if you are travelling, so I tend to make a big batch when I am doing them, and fill up all nine trays of the dehydrator. They are a fantastic substitute for bags of crisps, which have no health benefits whatsoever, and they contain wonderful nori, full of minerals which your bones will love. Stored in an airtight container, they will probably last a month, but in my house I have never had the chance to find out because they always get eaten much faster than that!

2 cups raw almonds, soaked overnight, with or without skins removed, rinsed and drained
2 cups raw sunflower seeds, soaked overnight, rinsed and drained
4 sticks celery, chopped
1 red pepper, destalked and seeds removed, chopped
2 tablespoons tahini
1 handful fresh parsley, chopped
1 handful fresh coriander, chopped
2 tablespoons lemon or lime juice
2 tablespoons (or more to taste) Bragg's Liquid Aminos or tamari
½-1 cup filtered water
2-3 teaspoons garam masala or curry powder
½ teaspoon cayenne pepper
Raw nori sheets

- Coarsely chop the almonds and sunflower seeds in the food processor with the S-blade (the standard blade that comes with food processors). Gradually add some water with the machine running to give a paste-like consistency that will spread.

- Add the remaining ingredients and blend well until you have a smooth paste, of slightly thinner consistency than pâté. Taste – add more spices if you prefer a hotter taste.
- Lay a nori sheet out flat and spread some mixture over half of the sheet, quite thinly (less than ½ cm thick). Fold the other half over to make a nori sandwich and press down carefully. Some mixture might squidge out at the side – just remove this and use on the next nori sheet.
- Once you have your nori sandwich, with the long edge towards you, cut it in half front to back with scissors, to give two approximately square pieces. Cut each of these pieces into quarters to make small squares that are approximately one and a half inches (4 cm) square. Place these squares on a dehydrator tray with Teflex sheet in place.
- Continue to use the remainder of the mixture to make further nori 'sandwiches', which you cut into squares and place on the dehydrator trays.
- Dehydrate at 115°F for one to two hours, then reduce the temperature to 105°F and dehydrate for about 12 hours or overnight. Flip the squares over and leave in the dehydrator for a further four to five hours.
- Allow to cool before storing in an airtight container. Bet you can't eat just one!

Cheese substitute

Finding it hard to drop the dairy products? Once you've tried this cheese substitute you may end up wondering why you ever ate the cow-derived version. The same goes for the milks below.

200g macadamia nuts
1 tablespoon white miso

Juice of 1 lemon
2 cloves garlic
Pure water

- Place all ingredients except the water into a blender and blend well. Add water a little at a time until a smooth, spreadable consistency is achieved.
- Use this anywhere you would normally use regular cheese; for example, spread the 'cheese' down the centre of celery sticks and serve. This makes a great snack on a hot day, or a light starter/appetizer. If you don't like celery, the cheese can be used as a dip for crackers or crudités.

Milk

You can of course buy almond milk and rice milk in cartons (please avoid soya milk), but it is preferable to make your own, since it is delicious and totally unprocessed. There are two ways to do it, depending if you want the quick and easy way or the more labour-intensive (but possibly more satisfying) way.

Quick milk

1-2 tablespoons raw almond butter or brazil nut butter
250ml water
½ teaspoon vanilla powder or 1 teaspoon alcohol-free vanilla essence
Pinch of stevia, or a few drops of liquid stevia (optional)

- Combine all the ingredients in a blender and blend well.

Slow milk

1 cup raw nuts, soaked overnight, rinsed and drained (brazil nuts, almonds or pecans work well)
3–4 cups water

½ teaspoon vanilla powder or 1 teaspoon alcohol-free vanilla essence
Pinch of stevia, or a few drops of liquid stevia (optional)

- Blend the soaked nuts and water.
- Strain the blended mixture through a muslin bag to avoid the milk having a grainy texture if you like.
- Return the strained milk to the blender and add the vanilla and stevia if you're using it.
- If you have strained the milk, you can use the remaining nut solids for adding to biscuits, pâtés and anything that's destined for the dehydrator.

Appendix 1

Bone-building green juice recipe

For anyone seriously wishing to maximise their mineral intake, a daily green juice is a must.

This is usually taken for breakfast. If you are new to green juice, do persevere; it really will have whole-body benefits.

The best green juice for bone building consists of, per person:

Celery (4 sticks)
1 cucumber
1 large handful of sunflower greens
1 large handful of pea shoots
1 piece of turmeric root
1 tablespoon liquid blue-green algae
2 oz wheatgrass juice
A few stinging nettles, if available

We can also make additions. Personally I never tire of the above list, but do quite frequently add extras, such as:

Kale	adds extra protein and minerals
Lemon	adds alkalising minerals and gives a tang to the juice
Lime	for the same reasons as lemon above
Garlic	fantastic for general detoxification and great for

	the immune system (also contains germanium)
Ginger	anti-inflammatory, warming and has benefits for the circulation.

Appendix 2

Juice Plus studies

Juice Plus, as I have mentioned in several chapters of this book, is one of my favourite supplements, and I have personally used it for 20 years. It has whole-body benefits. Here is some research to back up my recommendations. You can order it worldwide via my personal website: www.juiceplus.co.uk/+mt016459.

Juice PLUS+® delivers key phytonutrients that are absorbed by the body

Investigators at the University of South Carolina,[1] Tokyo Women's Medical University[2] and the Medical University of Vienna[3] studied the bioavailability (absorption by the body) of select nutrients found in Juice PLUS+® and concluded that Juice PLUS+® effectively increases antioxidant nutrients and folate. Other published studies have also shown various phytonutrients in Juice PLUS+® are bioavailable. These studies were conducted by independent researchers from the Georgetown/UCLA,[4] University of Sydney in Australia,[5] King's College in London,[6] Brigham Young University,[7] the University of Arizona,[8] the University of Florida,[9] and the University of Texas Health Science Center.[10]

Juice PLUS+® reduces oxidative stress

Several of these studies which included various aspects of nutrient bioavailability[1,2,6,9,10] also reported improved antioxidant enzyme levels, plasma antioxidant capacity and reduced lipid peroxides, a key indicator of oxidative stress. In addition, researchers at the Medical University of Graz, Austria[11,12] and the University of North Carolina, Greensboro[13,14] found that Juice PLUS+® Fruit, Vegetable and Vineyard Blends together were effective in reducing a marker for oxidative stress associated with aerobic exercise.

Juice PLUS+® can positively influence several markers of systemic inflammation in healthy people

Chronic inflammation is common. Emerging science is identifying different markers of generalised inflammation, even in otherwise healthy people. Published clinical research from the University of South Carolina[1] demonstrated Juice PLUS+® reduces several of these markers.

Juice PLUS+® helps maintain a healthy immune system and DNA integrity

Good nutrition is important for the normal function of the immune system and healthy DNA. Published clinical research indicated that Juice PLUS+® supports several measures of immune function – in law school students at the University of Florida[9] and in elderly people in a study conducted at the University of Arizona.[8] A study of healthcare professionals at Charité University Medical Centre in Berlin,[15] Germany, reported Juice PLUS+® use over the cold winter months resulted in a 20 per cent reduction in moderate/severe symptom days.

Studies conducted have shown a reduction in DNA damage after taking Juice PLUS+® in the law students at the University of Florida[9] and in an elderly population at Brigham Young University.[7]

Juice PLUS+® positively impacts several key indicators of cardiovascular wellness

Studies have been carried out into the effect of Juice PLUS+® on several markers of heart and vascular health.

Homocysteine is an amino acid that is found in the blood. Maintaining healthy homocysteine levels is thought to be important for the heart and cardiovascular system. A clinical study at the University of Sydney in Australia[5] reported a reduction in homocysteine levels – even though the levels of the Australian subjects were already within an acceptable range. Researchers in Foggia, Italy[16] also found a reduction of homocysteine levels in subjects with elevated levels of homocysteine.

Researchers at the University of Maryland School of Medicine[17] found that subjects who consumed Juice PLUS+® were better able to maintain the normal elasticity of arteries, even after a high-fat meal.

Investigators at Vanderbilt University School of Medicine[18] monitored several measures of vascular health in a low-risk population who took Juice PLUS+® for two years and noted various improvements with no adverse side effects.

Additional published results

Two pilot studies – one on the role of Juice PLUS+® in pregnancy health[19] and one on the effect of Juice PLUS+® on oxidative stress in smokers[20] – are now being followed up with placebo-controlled double-blind clinical trials.

References

1. Jin Y, et al. 'Systemic inflammatory load in humans is suppressed by consumption of two formulations of dried, encapsulated juice concentrate.' *Molecular Nutrition & Food Research* 2010; 54, 1-9.

2. Kawashima A, et al. 'Four week supplementation with mixed fruit and vegetable juice concentrates increased protective serum antioxidants and folate and decreased plasma homocysteine in Japanese subjects.' *Asia Pacific Journal of Clinical Nutrition* 2007; 16(3): 411-421.
3. Kiefer I, et al. 'Supplementation with mixed fruit and vegetable juice concentrates increased serum antioxidants and folate in healthy adults.' *Journal of the American College of Nutrition* 2004; 23(3): 205-211.
4. Wise JA, et al. 'beta-carotene and alpha-tocopherol in healthy overweight adults; depletion kinetics are correlated with adiposity.' *International Journal of Food Science and Nutrition* 2009; 60(S3): 65-75.
5. Samman S, et al. 'A mixed fruit and vegetable concentrate increases plasma antioxidant vitamins and folate and lowers plasma homocysteine in men.' *Journal of Nutrition* 2003; 133(7): 2188-2193.
6. Leeds AR, et al. 'Availability of micronutrients from dried, encapsulated fruit and vegetable preparations: a study in healthy volunteers.' *Journal of Human Nutrition and Dietetics* 2000; 13(1): 21-27.
7. Smith MJ, et al. 'Supplementation with fruit and vegetable extracts may decrease DNA damage in the peripheral lymphocytes of an elderly population.' *Nutrition Research* 1999; 19(10): 1507-1518.
8. Inserra PF, et al. 'Immune function in elderly smokers and nonsmokers improves during supplementation with fruit and vegetable extracts.' *Integrative Medicine* 1999; 2(1): 3-10.
9. Nantz MP, et al. 'Immunity and antioxidant capacity in humans is enhanced by consumption of a dried, encapsulated fruit and vegetable juice concentrate.' *Journal of Nutrition* 2006; 136(10): 2606-2610.
10. Wise JA, et al. 'Changes in plasma carotenoid, alpha-tocopherol, and lipid peroxide levels in response to supplementation

with concentrated fruit and vegetable extracts: a pilot study.' *Current Therapeutic Research* 1996; 57(6): 445-4619.

11. Lamprecht M, et al. 'Several indicators of oxidative stress, immunity, and illness improved in trained men consuming an encapsulated juice powder concentrate for 28 weeks.' *Journal of Nutrition* 2007; 137(12): 2737-2741.
12. Lamprecht M, et al. 'Protein modification responds to exercise intensity and antioxidant supplementation.' *Medicine & Science in Sports & Exercise* 2009; 41(1): 155-163.
13. Bloomer RJ, et al. 'Oxidative stress response to aerobic exercise: comparison of antioxidant supplements.' *Medicine & Science in Sports & Exercise* 2006; 38 (6): 1098-1105.
14. Goldfarb AH, et al. Effects of a Fruit/Berry/Vegetable supplement on muscle function and oxidative stress.' *Medicine and Science in Sports and Exercise* 2010 [ePub ahead of print].
15. Roll S, et al. 'Reduction of common cold symptoms by encapsulated juice powder concentrate of fruits and vegetables: a randomized, double-blind, placebo-controlled trial.' *British Journal of Nutrition* 2011; 105, 118-122.
16. Panunzio MF, et al. 'Supplementation with fruit and vegetable concentrate decreases plasma homocysteine levels in a dietary controlled trial.' *Nutrition Research* 2003; 23(9): 1221-1228.
17. Plotnick GD, et al. 'Effect of supplemental phytonutrients on impairment of the flow-mediated brachial artery vasoactivity after a single high-fat meal.' *Journal of the American College of Cardiology* 2003; 41(10): 1744-1749.
18. Houston MC, et al. 'Juice powder concentrate and systemic blood pressure, progression of coronary artery calcium and antioxidant status in hypertensive subjects: a pilot study.' *eCAM* 2007; 4(4): 455-462.
19. Odom CD, et al. 'Phytonutrients may decrease obstetric complications; a retrospective study.' *Journal of the American Nutraceutical Association* 2006; 9(1): 23-27.
20. Bamonti F, et al. 'Increased free malondialdehyde

concentrations in smokers normalise with a mixed fruit and vegetable juice concentrate; a pilot study.' *Clinical Chemistry and Laboratory Medicine* 2006; 44(4): 391-395.

Hospitals and universities that investigated or are investigating Juice PLUS+®

Brigham Young University, USA
Charité University, Berlin, Germany
Georgetown University, USA
King's College, London, England
Medical University of Graz, Austria
Medical University of Vienna, Austria
Tokyo Women's Medical University, Japan
University of Arizona, USA
University of Birmingham, England
University of California, Los Angeles, USA
University of Florida, USA
University of Maryland School of Medicine, USA
University of Milan, Italy
University of Mississippi Medical Center, USA
University of North Carolina-Greensboro, USA
University of South Carolina, USA
University of Sydney, Australia
University of Texas Health Science Center, USA
University of Texas/MD Anderson, USA
University of Würzburg, Germany
Vanderbilt University School of Medicine, USA
Wake Forest University, USA (with the NCI-National Institutes of Health)
Yale University-Griffin Hospital Prevention Research Center, USA

Resources

Living food centres and retreats

Hippocrates Health Institute: based in Florida, and run by Drs Brian and Anna-Maria Clement, Hippocrates offers a complete life change programme based on living foods. Many guests have been able to successfully rebuild their bone density by following the regime taught here. See www.hippocratesinst.org.

A retreat which I co-run in Gloucestershire, UK: www.rawfoodretreat.eu

Equipment and juicers

The Fresh Network: a one-stop shop for everything related to the living foods lifestyle. I recommend taking out a subscription to their quarterly e-magazine *Get Fresh*. www.fresh-network.com. You can also access the Fresh Network via the link from the shop page of my website: www.therawfoodscientist.com/Shop.htm.

Wholistic Health Direct/Wholistic Research Company: for a wide range of juicers and other equipment for a healthy lifestyle – www.wholisticresearch.com.

Home delivery of sprouts and wheatgrass for juicing

Aconbury Sprouts: next-day delivery of organically grown wheatgrass, sunflower greens, pea greens and all the seeds and grain you will need for growing your own indoor greens.

www.wheatgrass-uk.com.

My website

For details of the services I offer, including private and group consultations:

www.therawfoodscientist.com.

References

Introduction

1. Papadimitropoulos EA, Coyte PC, Josse RG, Greenwood CE. Current and projected rates of hip fracture in Canada. *Canadian Medical Association Journal* 1997; 158: 870-871.

Chapter 1

1. Johnell O, Kanis JA. An estimate of the worldwide prevalence and disability associated with osteoporotic fractures. *Osteoporosis International* 2006; 17: 1726.
2. Kanis JA. *World Health Organisation Technical Report, University of Sheffield, UK* 2007: 66.
3. EFFO and NOF. Who are candidates for prevention and treatment for osteoporosis? *Osteoporosis International 1997; 7: 1.*
4. Johnell O, Kanis JA. An estimate of the worldwide prevalence and disability associated with osteoporotic fractures. *Osteoporosis International* 2006; 17: 1726.
5. Melton LJ, Atkinson EJ, O'Connor MK, et al. (1998) Bone density and fracture risk in men. *Journal of Bone and Mineral Research* 13:1915; Melton LJ, Chrischilles EA, Cooper C, et al (1992) Perspective. How many women have osteoporosis? *Journal of Bone and Mineral Research* 7: 1005.

Chapter 2

1. Gross TS, Akeno N, Clemens TL, Komarova S, Srinivasan S, Weimer DA, Mayorov S. Osteocytes upregulate HIF-1κ in response to acute disuse and oxygen deprivation. *Journal of Applied Physiology* 2001; 90(6): 2514-2512.

2. Adams J, Fantner GE, Fisher LW, Hansma PK. Molecular energy dissipation in nanoscale networks of dentin matrix protein 1 is strongly dependent on ion valence. *Nanotechnology* 2008; 19: 384008.
3. Hansma PK, Fantner GE, Kindt JH, Thurner PJ, Schitter G, Turner PJ, Udwin SF, Finch MM. Sacrificial bonds in the interfibrillar matrix of bone. *Journal of Musculoskeletal and Neuronal Interactions* 2005; 5(4): 313-315.
4. Source: www.iofbonehealth.org/facts-statistics
5. Dalzell N, Kaptoge S, Morris N, et al. Bone micro-architecture and determinants of strength in the radius and tibia: age-related changes in a population based study of normal adults measured with high-resolution pQCT. *Osteoporosis International* 2009; 20(10): 1683-1694.
6. www.shef.ac.uk/FRAX.
7. Milovanovic P, Rakocevic Z, Djonic D, Zivkovic V, Hahn M, Nikolic S, Amling M, Busse, B, Djuric M. Nano-structural, compositional and micro-architectural signs of cortical bone fragility at the superolateral femoral neck in elderly hip fracture patients vs. healthy aged controls. *Experimental Gerontology* 2014; 55: 19-28.
8. Diez-Perez A, Güerri R, Nogues X, Cáceres E, Peña, MJ, Mellibovsky L, Randall C, Bridges D, Weaver JC, Proctor A. Microindentation for in vivo measurement of bone tissue mechanical properties in humans. *Journal of Bone and Mineral Research* 2010; 25: 1877-1885.

Chapter 3

1. Frassetto LA, Todd KM, Morris C, Jr et al. Worldwide incidence of hip fracture in elderly women: relation to consumption of animal and vegetable foods. *Journal of Gerontology* 2000; 55: M585-M592.
2. Ho SC. Body measurements, bone mass and fractures: does the East differ from the West? *Journal of Clinical Orthopaedics and Related Research* 1996; 323: 75-80.
3. Seiquer I, Delgado-Andrade C, Haro A, Navarro MP. Assessing the effects of severe heat treatment of milk on calcium bioavailability: in vitro and in vivo studies. *Journal of Dairy Science* 2010; 93(12): 5635-5643. doi: 10.3168/jds.2010-3469.
4. Lanou AJ, Berkow SE, Barnard ND. Calcium, Dairy Products, and Bone Health in Children and Young Adults: A Re-evaluation of the Evidence. *Pediatrics* 2005; 115(3): 736-743.
5. Keon J. The Real Truth About Health Conference, New York: January 2014.
6. Chan JM, Stampfer MJ, Ma J, et al. Insulin-like Growth Factor-1 (IGF-1) and IGF binding protein-3 as predictors of advanced-stage prostate cancer. *Journal of the National Cancer Institute* 2002; 94: 1099-1109.

7. Diehl H. The Real Truth About Health Conference, New York: January 2014
8. Karjalainen J, Martin JM, Knip M, et al. A bovine albumin peptide as a possible trigger of insulin-dependent Diabetes Mellitus. *New England Journal of Medicine* 1992; 327: 302-307.
9. McDougall J, Bruce B, Spiller G, Westerdahl J, McDougall M. Effects of a very low-fat, vegan diet in subjects with rheumatoid arthritis. *Journal of Alternative and Complementary Medicine* 2002; 8(1): 71-75.

Chapter 4

1. Buclin T, Cosma M, Appenzeller M, Jacquet A-F, Décosterd LA, Biollaz J, Burckhardt P. Diet Acids and Alkalis Influence Calcium Retention in Bone. *Osteoporosis International* 2001: 12(6): 493-499.
2. Gaby AR. Preventing and Reversing Osteoporosis. Thailand: Prima Publishing; 1994.
3. Kanis JA, Johnell O, Oden A, JohanssonH, et al. Smoking and fracture risk: a meta-analysis. *Osteoporosis International* 2005; 16(2): 155-162.
4. Bushinsky DA. Acidosis and bone. *Mineral and Electrolyte Metabolism.* 1994; 20(1-2): 40-52.
5. Bushinsky DA, Sprague SM, Hallegot P, Girod C, Chabala JM, Levi-Setti R. Effects of aluminum on bone surface ion composition. *Journal of Bone and Mineral Research* 1995; 10(12): 1988-1997.
6. Søgaard AJ, Meyer HE, Emaus N, Grimnes G, Gjesdal CG, Forsmo S, Schei B, Tell GS. Cohort profile: Norwegian Epidemiologic Osteoporosis Studies (NOREPOS). *Scandinavian Journal of Public Health* 2014; 2: pii: 1403494814551858.
7. Watanabe T, Kishikawa Y. Degradation of myocardiac myosin and creatine kinase in rats given alkaline ionized water. *Journal of Veterinary Medical Science* 1998; 60(2): 245-250.

Chapter 5

1. Wachsman A, Bernstein DS. Diet and osteoporosis. *Journal of the American Geriatric Society* 1982; 30: 613.
2. Abelow BJ, Holford TR, Insogna KL. Cross-cultural association between dietary animal protein and hip fracture: a hypothesis. *Calcified Tissue International* 1992; 50: 14-18.
3. Breslau NA, Brinkley L, Hill KD et al. Relationship of animal protein-rich diet to kidney stone formation and calcium metabolism. *Journal of Clinical and Endocrinology and Metabolism* 1998; 66: 140-146.
4. Frassetto LA, Todd KM, Morris C, Jr, et al. Worldwide incidence of hip fracture in elderly women: relation to consumption of animal and vegetable foods. *Journal of Gerontology* 2000; 55: M585-M592.

Chapter 6

1. Gordon GG, Lieber CS. Alcohol, hormones, and metabolism. In: Lieber CS (Ed) *Medical and Nutritional Complications of Alcoholism.* New York: Plenum Publishing Corp, 1992: 55-90.
2. Dandona P et al. Glucose Challenge Stimulates Reactive Oxygen Species (ROS) Generation by Leucocytes. *Journal of Clinical Endocrinology and Metabolism* 2000; 85: 2970-2973.
3. Ray M. *From Here to Longevity*. Seattle, USA: Shining Star Publishing; 2002.
4. Schretlen DJ, Inscore AB, Jinnah HA, et al. Serum Uric Acid and Cognitive Function in Community-Dwelling Older Adults. *Neuropsychology* 2007; 21(1): 136-140.
5. Dizdaroglu M, Jaruga P, Birincioglu M, Rodriguez H. Free radical-induced damage to DNA: mechanisms and measurement. *Free Radical Biology and Medicine* 2002; 32(11): 1102-1115.
6. Yang Q, Zhang Z, Gregg EW, et al. Added Sugar Intake and Cardiovascular Diseases Mortality Among US Adults. *JAMA Internal Medicine* 2014; 174(4): 516-524.
7. Rasheed P, Al-Sowielem LS. Prevalence and predictors of premenstrual syndrome among college-aged women in Saudi Arabia. *Annals of Saudi Medicine* 2003; 23(6): 381-387.

Chapter 7

1. Walker ARP, Walker BF, Richardson BD. Metacarpal bone dimensions in young and aged South African Bantu consuming a diet low in calcium. *Postgraduate Medical Journal* 1971; 47: 320-325.
2. Michaëlsson K, Melhus H, Bellocco R, Wolk A. Dietary calcium and vitamin D intake in relation to osteoporotic fracture risk. *Bone* 2003; 32(6): 694-703.
3. Kervran LC. *Preuves en Biologie de Transmutations à Faible Énergie.* Paris: Maloine; 1975.
4. Recker RR, Davis KM, Hinders SM et al. Bone gain in young adult women. *Journal of the American Medical Association* 1992; 268: 2403-2408.
5. Sellmeyer DE, Stone KL, Sebastian A, et al. A high ratio of dietary animal to vegetable protein increases the rate of bone loss and the risk of fracture in post-menopausal women. *American Journal of Clinical Nutrition* 2001; 73: 118-122.
6. 9. Adluri RS, Zhan L, Bagchi M, Maulik N, Maulik G. Comparative effects of a novel plant-based calcium supplement with two common calcium salts on proliferation and mineralization in human osteoblast cells. *Molecular and Cellular Biochemistry* 2010; 340(1-2): 73-80.

7. Marone PA, Yasmin T, Gupta RC, Bagchi M. Safety and toxicological evaluation of AlgaeCal (AC), a novel plant-based calcium supplement. *Toxicology Mechanisms and Methods* 2010; 20(6): 334-344.
8. Chakraborti S, Chakraborti T, Mandal M, Mandal A, Das S, Ghosh S. Protective role of magnesium in cardiovascular diseases: a review. *Molecular and Cellular Biochemistry* 2002; 238(1-2): 163-179.

Chapter 8

1. Zittermann A. Magnesium deficit – overlooked cause of low vitamin D status? *BioMed Central Medicine* 2013; 11: 229. doi:10.1186/1741-7015-11-229
2. Liebscher DH, Liebscher DE. About the Misdiagnosis of Magnesium Deficiency. *Journal of the American College of Nutrition* 2004; 23(6): 730S-731S.
3. Keen CL, Zidenberg-Cherr S. Manganese. In: Ziegler EE, Filer LJ (Eds). *Present Knowledge in Nutrition, 7th ed.* Washington DC, USA: ILSI Press; 1996: 334-343.
4. Nielsen FH, Hunt CD, Mullen LM, Hunt JR. Effect of dietary boron on mineral, estrogen, and testosterone metabolism in postmenopausal women. *FASEB J* 1987; 1: 394-397.
5. Atik OS. Zinc and senile osteoporosis. *Journal of the American Geriatric Society* 1983; 31: 790-791.
6. Shankar AH, Prasad AS. Zinc and immune function: the biological basis of altered resistance to infection. *American Journal of Clinical Nutrition* 1998; 68(2 Suppl): 447S-463S.
7. Price CT, Koval KJ, Langford JR. Silicon: A Review of Its Potential Role in the Prevention and Treatment of Postmenopausal Osteoporosis. *International Journal of Endocrinology* 2013, Article ID 316783.

Chapter 9

1. Falch JA. 1998. Low levels of serum ascorbic acid in elderly patients with hip fracture. *Scandinavian Journal of Clinical and Laboratory Investigation* 1998; 58(3): 225-228.
2. Yamaguchi M (2006). Regulatory mechanism of food factors in bone metabolism and prevention of osteoporosis. *Yakugaku Zasshi* 2006; 126(11): 1117–1137.
3. Feskanich D, Weber P, Willett WC, et al. Vitamin K intake and hip fractures in women: a prospective study. *American Journal of Clinical Nutrition* 1999; 69(1): 74-79.
4. Weaver CM. Diet, Microbiome and Bone Health. American Society for Bone Mineral Research Conference 2014: Meet the Professor discussion.

5. McLean RR, Jacques PF, Selhub J, et al. Homocysteine as a predictive factor for hip fracture in older persons. *New England Journal of Medicine* 2004; 350: 2042-2049.
6. Momken I, Stevens L, Bergouignan A, Desplanches D, Rudwill F, et al. Resveratrol prevents the wasting disorders of mechanical unloading by acting as a physical exercise mimetic in the rat. *The Federation of American Societies for Experimental Biology Journal Strasbourg, France:* Institut Pluridisciplinaire Hubert Curien (IPHC), Université de Strasbourg; 1998.
7. Chen JR, Lazarenko OP, Kang J et al. Dietary-induced serum phenolic acids promote bone growth via p38 MAPK/B-catenin canonical Wnt signalling. *Journal of Bone and Mineral Research* 2010; 25(11): 2399-2411.
8. Devareddy L, Hooshmand S, Collins JK, Lucas EA, Chai SC, Arjmandi BH. Blueberry prevents bone loss in ovariectomised rat model of postmenopausal osteoporosis. *Journal of Nutritional Biochemistry* 2008; 19(10): 694-699.
9. Aggarwal BB, Shishodia S. Suppression of the nuclear factor kappaB activation pathway by spice-derived phytochemicals: reasoning for seasoning. *Proceedings of the National Academy of Sciences* 2004; 1030: 434-441.
10. Shishodia S, Sethi G, Aggarwal BB. Curcumin: getting back to the roots. *Proceedings of the National Academy of Sciences 2005;* 1056: 206-217.
11. Langman CB. Calcitrol metabolism during chronic metabolic acidosis. *Seminars in Nephrology* 1989; 9: 65-71.
12. Byrne PM, Freaney R, McKenna MJ. Vitamin D supplementation in the elderly: review of safety and effectiveness of different regimes. *Calcified Tissue International* 1995; 56: 518-520.
13. Fontana L, Shew JL, Holloszy JO, Villareal DT. Low bone mass in subjects on a long-term raw vegetarian diet. *Archives of Internal Medicine* 2005; 165: 1-6.
14. Byers T. Anticancer Vitamins du Jour—The ABCED's So Far. *American Journal of Epidemiology* 2010; 172(1): 1–3.
15. McLeod JG, Hammond SR, Hallpike JF. Epidemiology of multiple sclerosis in Australia. With NSW and SA survey results. *Medical Journal of Australia* 1994; 160: 117-122.
16. Chan JM, Stampfer MJ, Ma J, et al. Insulin-like growth factor-1 (IGF-1) and IGF binding protein-3 as predictors of advanced-stage prostate cancer. *Journal of the National Cancer Institute* 2002; 94: 1099-1109.
17. Lappe JM, et al. Vitamin D and calcium supplementation reduces cancer risk: results of a randomized trial. *American Journal of Clinical Nutrition* 2007; 85: 1568–1591.

Chapter 10

1. Gupta S, Hrishikeshvan HJ, Sehajpal PK. Spirulina protects against Rosiglitazone induced osteoporosis in insulin resistant rats. *Diabetes Research and Clinical Practice* 2009; 4.
2. Caudarella R, Vescini F, Rizzoli E, Francucci CM. Salt intake, hypertension, and osteoporosis. *Journal of Endocrinological Investigation* 2009; 32(4 Suppl): 15-20.
3. Rico, H. Alcohol and bone disease. *Alcohol and Alcoholism* 1990; 25(4): 345-352.
4. McClung MR, et al. Romosozumab in postmenopausal women with low bone mineral density. *New England Journal of Medicine* 2014; 370(5): 412-420.

Chapter 11

1. Chyun YS, Kream BE, Raisz LG. Cortisol decreases bone formation by inhibiting periosteal cell proliferation. *Endocrinology* 1984; 114(2): 477-480.
2. Levine G. In: *Circulation* May 9, 2013.
3. Rosano GM, Panina G. Oestrogens and the heart. *Therapie* 1999; 54(3): 381-385.
4. Scientific American's Updated Medicine Text, 1991.
5. Burrows M, Nevill AM, Bird S, Simpson D. Physiological factors associated with low bone mineral density in female endurance runners. *British Journal of Sports Medicine* 2003; Feb; 37(1): 67-71.
6. Villareal DT, Holloszy JO, Kohrt WM. Effects of DHEA replacement on bone mineral density and body composition in elderly women and men. *Clinical Endocrinology* 2000; 53(5): 561-568.
7. Landin-Wilhelmsen K, Nilsson A, Bosaeus I, Bengtsson BA. Growth hormone increases bone mineral content in postmenopausal osteoporosis: a randomized placebo-controlled trial. *Journal of Bone and Mineral Research* 2003; 18(3): 393-405.
8. Franklin JA, et al. Long-term thyroxine treatment and bone mineral density. *Lancet* 1992; 340: 9-13.

Chapter 12

1. Shenoy S. Exercise in osteoporosis *British Journal of Sports Medicine* 2010; 44 (Suppl 1): i3-i3.
2. Borer KT. Physical activity in the prevention and amelioration of osteoporosis in women: interaction of mechanical, hormonal and dietary factors. *Sports Medicine* 2005; 35: 779-830.
3. Kohrt M, Bloomfield SA, Little KD, et al. Physical activity and bone

health. Position stand of the American College of Sports Medicine. *Medicine and Science in Sports and Exercise* 2004; 36: 1985-1996.

4. Chilibeck PD, Sale DG, Webber CE. Exercise and bone mineral density. *Sports Medicine* 1995; 19: 103-122.

Index

Index